sleep rituals

100 PRACTICES FOR A DEEP AND PEACEFUL SLEEP

jennifer williamson

Adams Media

New York   London   Toronto   Sydney   New Delhi

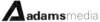

Adams Media
An Imprint of Simon & Schuster, Inc.
57 Littlefield Street
Avon, Massachusetts 02322

First Adams Media hardcover edition January 2019

ADAMS MEDIA and colophon are trademarks of Simon & Schuster.

For information about special discounts for bulk purchases, please contact Simon & Schuster Special Sales at 1-866-506-1949 or business@simonandschuster.com.

The Simon & Schuster Speakers Bureau can bring authors to your live event. For more information or to book an event contact the Simon & Schuster Speakers Bureau at 1-866-248-3049 or visit our website at www.simonspeakers.com.

Interior design by Katrina Machado
Interior images © Getty Images/sumkinn, Mila_1989, Anatartan

Manufactured in the United States of America

10 9 8 7 6 5 4 3 2 1

Library of Congress Cataloging-in-Publication Data has been applied for.

ISBN 978-1-5072-0952-3
ISBN 978-1-5072-0953-0 (ebook)

CONTENTS

INTRODUCTION

Sleep is a time to heal, a time of peace, a time when every heavy thing from your day falls away so you can rest your body and recharge your soul. Indeed, the most profound gift of a restful sleep is the way you are strengthened from within: it makes life feel *lighter*. The rituals in this book will help you enter the deep, nourishing stages of sleep that make it possible for your total well-being to blossom.

In this accessible guide to a restful slumber, you will learn how to turn your mind, body, and space into an ideal sanctuary for sleep. No more rushing from task to task and hoping your brain shuts off on command—*Sleep Rituals* shows you how to slow down and explore the qualitative difference between day and night. Using these one hundred easy and peaceful rituals—personal practices you treat with intention—you'll be able to tune in to your body and your surroundings and tune out superficial noise and worry, clearing space in your mind for sleep. Each restorative practice in this book, whether it calls for a cup of tea or therapeutic touch, serves as a chance to get to know (and enjoy) yourself better. The intimacy of that *self*-exploration is a divine relaxation.

Expect more than a collection of habits in this book—after all, healing and renewal require something richer than mindless repetition. Rituals enhance your ability to sweeten your life through something as simple as how you prepare for sleep. You're both harnessing your relationship with yourself and your relationship with sleep to make joy, creativity, and well-being a daily reality. You can most certainly expect to wake up, work, play, love, give, and grow more gracefully—all because you've given yourself the essential gift of real rest.

CHAPTER 1

SETTING THE TONE

For most adults, 7–9 hours of sleep are essential for building emotional resilience, physical stamina, mental clarity, creative capacity, and healthy relationships. Your quality of life depends on making sleep a priority. While an upheaval in lifestyle is not necessarily the key to better sleep, a tender loving tweak in your perspective may be.

Mastering the subtle art of loving yourself to sleep requires you to treat the mundane like it matters, too, because it's the foundation any successful ritual rests on. A beautiful ritual practice creates the conditions necessary for sleep, but don't dismiss the routine that breathes consistency into your life. This includes going to bed and waking up at the same time each day and also the ways that you go about making that a reality. Attended to with care, even something as casual as dimming the lights becomes an invocation for sleep. Sleep loves this kind of consistent, detail-oriented, respectful attention.

You don't need to change everything all at once. Start with one small change at a time. Treat this prep time with the same devotion that makes a ritual so powerful. Pay attention to the subtleties of your transition from day to night. If you start here, tonight, with the quiet pact to honor the little things, you have already begun the healing work.

TURNING THE BEDROOM INTO A SANCTUARY

Better sleep requires a bedroom that is set up for sleep—and only sleep. With today's constant flow of information and stimulation, it is more crucial than ever to sanction off a space where you can disconnect from stress and reconnect with peace. Treating your bedroom like the most sacred space in your home is one of the most revolutionary decisions you can make—you'll be spending about one-third of the rest of your life here. Let this be a pleasurable place to come home to. Design it with comfort, security, restoration, and sensuality in mind. This one conscious act of self-care will breathe harmony into all areas of your life.

Creating a serene bedroom begins by declaring the purpose of this space: rest, intimacy, and perhaps contemplation. Set your own personal intention for the bedroom by choosing a word or phrase that depicts what this space is going to be used for from now on. For instance, you might declare something like "This is where I love, rest, and dream." Every time you walk into your room, reaffirm its purpose.

You will need to set a healthy and firm boundary in order to turn your bedroom into a space that reflects your intentions—and keeps unharmonious energies out. Consider the following suggestions to help you get into the mindset of boundary setting:

- ★ Hang a doorknob tag that affirms your intention, such as "Healing in progress," "No shoes allowed," or "Only sacred vibes here."

- ★ Designate bedtime apparel. Sleeping in the same clothes you wore today sends mixed messages. Select breathable clothing dedicated to sleep: breezy nightdresses, cozy pajamas, oversized T-shirts.

- ★ Associate your bed with fatigue. Avoid paperwork, news, email, text messages, games, arguments, and any stimulating or stressful activities. Get out of bed and perform some rituals if you have trouble falling asleep or staying asleep, rather than tossing and turning.

- ★ Share your bed with care. If pets are taking over, it may be time to reclaim your space (this may be one of the harder decisions you make, but whatever you decide, decide consciously). If it's more of a partner thing, invest in a bigger (quality) mattress where you can both sleep in comfort.

- ★ Eliminate distractions. Remove the television, computer, bills, and exercise equipment. If these items must stay, unplug and create a barrier using a lightweight folding screen or beautiful fabric hung from a curtain rod or draped over items.

- ★ Ban technology. Disengage from the world by turning off all electronic devices and/or leaving them in another room. At the very least, put them on airplane mode. There is a time and a place for everything under the sun: stimulation jives with the sun; restoration is the moon's specialty. Live by nature's rhythms and give your screen some space.

THE FOUNDATIONS OF SLEEP: TEMPERATURE, LIGHTING, AND SOUND

With boundaries in place, your bedroom will naturally begin to ripen with intention over time. To usher that process along, there are three elements you will want to experiment with, for the sake of uninterrupted sleep: temperature, lighting, and sound. When properly attended to, these pillars of sleep will signal to your brain that it's time to rest and your body will intuitively begin to unwind. Returning to a cool, dark, and quiet room after your rituals is a lullaby for your entire system.

TEMPERATURE

Just like Mother Nature, your body naturally lowers its temperature in the evening. The cooler you become, the easier sleep can come. Keep your bedroom temperature somewhere around 65°F to initiate the body's progression into sleep and ensure that you are not woken by being too hot or too cold.

To maintain an optimal sleeping temperature, you can:

★ Set your bedroom thermostat to automatically adjust before bedtime.

★ Open windows for improved circulation.

★ Bring in a fan (make sure it's not blowing directly on you).

★ Use a cooling pillow or mattress pad.

★ Choose bedding and sleepwear to suit the season: thicker in the winter, lighter in the summer.

★ Keep an extra blanket, slippers, socks, or a robe nearby to ease you out of bed in the morning.

LIGHTING

As the sun goes down, the dip in temperature coincides with darkness—another of nature's sleep tonics. The body's natural response to the setting sun is to produce the hormone melatonin, which brings about sleepiness, but bright light at night tells your brain to stop secreting melatonin because it's not time to sleep (the message: "the sun is still shining"). The steady stream of blue light emanating from screens is especially good at suppressing melatonin. This confusion leaves an obedient body prone to unhealthy sleep habits and chronic illness.

Love your body back to calm by embracing softer lighting in the evening and darkness at night. Reduce your exposure to bright lights at least 1–2 hours before bedtime and make a few adjustments to support a smoother transition into sleep, including:

★ Trade harsh overhead lighting for several smaller sources of light: Himalayan salt lamps, nightlights, strings of fairy lights, diffused lighting products, flickering candles, a fireplace.

★ Install a dimmer switch for instant dream appeal.

★ Invest in window coverings, such as blackout curtains, that can be pulled closed for a cocoon-like ambience after nightfall.

★ Keep an eye pillow on your nightstand.

★ Soften the glow of your alarm clock. Turn it away from you, put it under your bed or nightstand, or cover it with fabric.

★ Use amber-colored glasses that block blue light.

★ Use a nighttime filter on screens to emit a warmer, sleep-inducing hue. Blue light–blocking software exists if your device does not have this built-in functionality.

★ Declare digital freedom (if you haven't already). Set a lighthearted notification on your phone to remind you that it's time to put the technology away—"I need to rest" or "We need space"—and then stop using those devices that stimulate your brain. This includes cell phones, tablets, ereaders, laptops, computers, televisions, and video games.

SOUND

Being in right relationship to technology and nature's rhythms deepens your connection to life in this moment—where you're meant to be. Nighttime is about peace and quiet in the here and now, not disruptions, hence the third foundational element of sound sleep: sound.

Even while you sleep, your brain continues to register and process sounds. If complete silence isn't in the cards, creating a soothing environment with soft sounds that you personally enjoy gives you a better chance at sleeping through the night undisturbed by any sudden noises. Find what works for you:

★ Create a constant ambient sound with "colored" noises. Sound machines play white, pink, and brown noise that helps mask other potentially wakeful noises. White: static, fan, air purifier. Pink is often found in nature: steady rainfall, leaves rustling in the trees, waves lapping on the beach. Brown is more skewed toward lower frequencies: thunder, the low roaring of a waterfall.

- ★ Listen to podcasts or books on tape that are meant for relaxation and sleep. Keep the volume just barely audible and set a timer so the noise doesn't wake you up in the middle of the night.
- ★ Place a rolled-up towel at the base of your door to reduce sounds outside your bedroom.
- ★ Keep noise-canceling headphones or earplugs on your nightstand.
- ★ Replace rude awakenings (and the anticipation of a jolting alarm) with a sunlight alarm clock that wakes you gently.
- ★ Turn off notifications on all devices. Habitually responding to these sounds during the day means you're likely to respond to them while you're sleeping.
- ★ Turn off or remove wireless routers. Wi-Fi signals produce no detectable sound but they give off an invisible tone or pulsed frequency that might disturb sleep.

Your bedroom is cool, dark, and hushed, just as Mother Nature intended. With the core essentials in place, you can begin taking care of the heart of this space: the energy you grow and tend to here. Explore those sensory and feeling elements that welcome healing vibes and make rest seem as natural as the stars in the sky.

SURROUND YOURSELF WITH COMFORT

From the color of your walls to what's on your nightstand, surround yourself with the physical manifestations of comfort, peace, and sensuality. Ask yourself which items are conducive to a surrender to sleep and which tether you to the waking world. Choosing art, symbols, and objects that resonate with your intentions is both a creative act and a sacred practice. Ultimately, go with what inspires you and elicits a pleasant response. This space is yours, so it's about how *you* want to feel when you are here. A few thoughtful tweaks can make all the difference:

★ Trade crisp whites for warm neutral colors: beige, cream, super-soft gray. Bask in rich earth tones: pine, terra-cotta, cocoa. Replace bright colors with pale blues, dusty rose, muted greens, or lavender. Balance with deep accents like pomegranate and eggplant for a sensual touch.

★ Opt for natural, organic bedding materials like cotton or bamboo that feel luxurious. Sleep on an earthing sheet or mat to potentially reduce exposure to EMFs (electromagnetic fields). Use a weighted blanket for therapeutic comfort and a sense of protection.

★ Consider bed placement to support the flow of calm energy. Avoid placing in front of a window if possible. Place against a solid wall with a solid wood headboard or add large pillows behind you. Be as far away from the door as possible so you can see the whole room. Use a folding screen, curtains, or a piece of furniture to suggest protection from doors and adjoining rooms.

★ Select serene, romantic, or pleasant images and artwork, especially if seen from the bed. Avoid photos of others aside from your partner.

★ Remove or cover mirrors and other reflective surfaces at night to quiet the energy.

★ Celebrate your connection to the earth. Replace synthetic materials and fragrances with grounding gifts from nature:

thriving houseplants, wood, natural candles, pure essential oils, gemstones, etc.

★ Embrace curves. Soften corners by draping fabric over tables and dressers. Let leaves cascade over sharp edges. Cover ceiling beams with cloth. Avoid anything looming overhead.

★ Honor your nightstand. Keep a journal (for rituals, dream recall, or tracking sleep quality), oils and misters, poetry, or one or two crystals by your bedside: selenite for cleansing, rose quartz for emotional balancing, amethyst for intuition and dreaming, black tourmaline for grounding and protection.

Everything you are doing is transforming your bedroom into a blissful reflection of your intentions: loving, resting, dreaming. Thank yourself for creating a haven where you can come to be recharged and nourished from the ground up.

TIDYING UP WITH INTENTION

Take inventory of your entire living space. Close your eyes and bring to mind a few adjectives that capture the way you'd like to feel about each room. Set an intention for each room, just like you did with your bedroom. Open your eyes and compare notes.

There is a strong link between chaos in the home and chaos in the head. Thankfully, you can do something about the visual mess in order to tame the mental stress. Clearing away dust and distraction subconsciously calms overactive thoughts. No need to overwhelm yourself with what you find: doing just a little bit each night to honor the *space* in your space will do wonders for your state of mind (and your sleep).

Here is a menu, not a checklist, of ways you can move through your home with tender loving care, turning an otherwise heartless chore into a candid request for restoration and peace, inside and out:

★ Stack or put away laundry, mail, and papers with your adjectives and intentions for that room in mind.

★ Neaten your bed covers, bookshelves, and coffee tables as though you were tucking everything in for the night.

★ Organize clutter behind closed doors and underneath beds, accepting a deeper sense of control over your life.

★ Take out the trash and wash the dishes, imagining the residue of your day going out the door and flowing down the drain.

★ Sprinkle rugs with baking soda mixed with dried lavender flowers before vacuuming away stagnant energy held in the fibers.

★ Wrap your broom with ribbon and sweep away physical and energetic cobwebs and debris, making sure to sweep all entrances.

★ Let go of old, unworn, or unwanted items that don't delight, inspire, or serve you—letting any worn-out thought patterns, perceptions, or pain go with them. Throw them away or give them away to someone who might find more pleasure through them. This builds your awareness of your attachments so that you can start experimenting with the sweetness of release.

The act of putting away, throwing away, or giving away just one thing each night symbolizes your receptivity to something new. Imagine the inflow of fresh energy saturating the space you just made, setting the tone for the rituals to come.

PLANNING FOR TOMORROW

With a space ready to serve your favorite rituals and your best sleep, preparing for a good morning is one of the most practical things you can do tonight to show your future self some love. Planning ahead is a fruitful endeavor: an easier and less stressful morning sets you up for a happier day and improves your chances of coming home feeling fulfilled (rather than depleted). You are essentially organizing a series of seamless moments, which naturally creates ease in *this* moment. The benefits come full circle.

Ask yourself how you can help your future self. Rather than feeling energetically malnourished in the morning, get the good vibes flowing tonight. Just a few minutes of prep work now gives you that much more space to actually enjoy the beginning of a new day.

Consider the simple but space-giving things you could do each night to help yourself rise and shine tomorrow:

★ Take out everything you need to make breakfast and lunch. Fill a jar with ingredients for overnight oats or a make-ahead smoothie.

★ Plan and lay out your work and gym outfits. Iron if needed.

★ File papers and pack your bag. Save anything that's overly stressful, such as paying bills, for when the sun is shining.

★ Write down your intentions for how you want to feel tomorrow and what kind of energy you want to bring to your interactions. Contemplate what you will do in the morning to feel this way.

★ Make tomorrow's to-do list and then relax, knowing that your priorities are scheduled.

Taking care of tomorrow designates space for intimacy tonight.

SET YOURSELF UP FOR SUCCESSFUL SLEEP

After preparing for the morning, bring your attention back to the energy of this moment and this environment you've created for yourself. Praise the consistency of your routine for what it allows: an opening in time insulated from everywhere else, set aside for something sacred. Celebrate this possibility to perceive life in its fullest expression—in the *here* and *now*. Ritual is a way to ripen the evening hours, to make them more substantial. Through ritual you invite the present to prevail.

Since a deep and peaceful sleep is what you are here for, the rituals themselves should be soothing and restorative (energy attracts like energy), and they are. You are learning to relax before you rest; you are affirming your love of sleep as you approach it. It is about choosing ambience over excitement. It is about tuning out all that makes it impossible to hear and follow the rhythm of the moment. It is about pausing to contemplate having finished something of value. Leave the glow of the screen behind because the more you participate, the deeper the healing potential of the practice, and the deeper balance is restored. Rooting yourself in the present moment turns out to be real self-care.

Creating new sleep patterns requires more than a change of behavior; it requires a change of heart. Your intention is the heart of ritual and is what imbues the mundane with an element of the magical. For a successful ritual, you will want to bring your wholehearted focus and a sense of curiosity. There is a lot of feeling and intuition involved. Be conscious and deliberate as you engage with every subtle nuance and sensation that comes up. Ultimately, tapping into restful rhythms will prove itself an inward journey of recovery and discovery, wholeness and union.

Trust your intuition to guide you to the rituals that support you tonight. Say yes to what resonates. Keep a steady and sincere devotion to whichever rituals you feel drawn to mixing and matching (refer to this book's appendix for designing ritual sequences). Give your mind and body permission to learn how to fall asleep differently. With patience, your practice will begin to feel like second nature and an energetic sanctuary in time—what's missing when your mind is cluttered and your heart is closed.

Remember that your rituals will likely look different from other people's, even those you share a home with. This is about consulting your inner guidance system and learning to answer your own needs. Great self-care is custom, intuitive, and kind. As your needs change in accordance with the seasons of your life, your practice will likely change, growing richer and more meaningful. Take your time. Find your rhythm. It's as though you're following a delicious bread crumb trail; you are always encountering something else that resonates with you and brings you back home to your most peaceful self. Enjoy.

—— CHAPTER 2 ——

CLEANSING AND ELEVATING YOUR SPACE

Just as sweeping away dust bunnies from the past can leave you feeling mentally clear, attending to the energy of your space can positively alter your state of mind. Though invisible, energy is always present. You have likely sensed the heavy energy in a room after an argument or the cheerful energy following a visit from friends. Like a sponge, space can hold on to emotions, thoughts, and activities long after they have transpired—even a visibly beautiful home can feel *off*. Bring to mind those spaces that have felt comfortable and restorative. Tune in to that same energetic frequency because it's what this chapter is going to help you bask in for a better night's sleep.

Each ritual presented here is a slow melt into peace. You will address energetic debris tucked away in nooks and crannies, clearing away what feels stressful and stagnant so that calming energy can circulate freely. As you infuse your home with your intentions for peaceful sleep—and any sounds, scents, and sights that support you—your environment will begin to reflect how you want to feel. Through practice, your space will ripen into a place where healing and sleep come naturally.

Experiment with one ritual at a time as you create an atmosphere of restoration. However you choose to make your whole home feel like a sanctuary, consider dedicating a special space for your tools—incense, essential oils, candles, crystals, music, singing bowls, bells, and so on. You might even call this your altar and use this space for meditation, breathing, and yoga practices, bringing in blankets, cushions, and journals. Treat this room, corner of a room, tabletop, or drawer with respect. Let it be where you go for comfort, connection to the divine and yourself, and transportation into a blissful slumber.

Whenever you find yourself in this space you have created, your mind will automatically know that it's time to go inward. You won't just be coming home to a house; you will be coming home to yourself.

1. CREATING A SOOTHING SOUNDSCAPE

Music is vibrational medicine. Over the course of history, music has played an instrumental role in healing and transforming us spiritually and physically. Certain frequencies (the speed of a vibration) in particular are believed to produce biological changes that mirror the sleeping body: slowing heart rate and breathing, lowering blood pressure, and relaxing the muscles. This direct effect on your internal rhythms is why music is used to aid digestion, bolster mental and emotional health, boost immunity, promote trauma recovery, reduce pain, promote mindfulness, and induce quality sleep. Sound therapy is a practical approach to elevating your space into a nourishing, restful haven.

There is music to soothe, uplift, meditate, pray, and sleep. Choosing tonight's music is a personal preference—but since your body syncs with the vibrational frequency, slower rhythms are ideal for relaxation and sleep. Listen to your heart as you gather a library of songs (online or physical) and musical tools to enhance your whole being, and nearly every other ritual in this book:

★ Classical music (slow symphonies) has proven itself a proponent of improved sleep quality, but folk songs, blues, and jazz can generate the ambience you're listening for.

★ Peaceful nature sounds create an instant atmosphere of serenity: also called "pink noise," it's an alternative to "white noise" in the bedroom.

★ Celestial melodies are inherent in guided meditations, shamanic sound healing, and other meditative collaborations. Explore artists producing uplifting, spiritual music.

★ Binaural beats therapy (usually accompanied by headphones) intends to create a shift in consciousness by matching brain waves to specific, repetitive tones. Research before trying, as effects can vary.

★ Chanting helps revitalize and harmonize your space, inside and out. Gregorian chant or mystical Sanskrit chants can release ordinary thought patterns and cultivate an openness to the present moment.

To help break up stagnant energy and restore harmony to the home and body, you may also choose to use instruments—helpful in certain space clearing and blessing ceremonies in this chapter. Standing in the center of a room and then walking around its perimeter with your sound healing tool of choice disperses old energy in hard-to-reach areas. Choose metal or crystal singing bowls, drums, Tibetan bells, gongs, chimes, a pan and a spoon or simply your own two hands, clapping away the old and bringing in the new.

Accompanied by a subdued melody, the body, mind, heart, and soul experience deep tranquility, allowing the experience of sleep to unfold more naturally. With appreciation and attention, every breath becomes part of the music, every moment a chance for self-exploration and liberation, and your space: living poetry. Even sleep is part of the subtle dance.

2. DIFFUSING ESSENTIAL OILS

Essential oils are potent plant extracts sourced from various parts including leaves, petals, stems, roots, bark, seeds, and fruits. These fragrant essences have long been used to soothe the body and mind, open the heart, and encourage restful sleep. Diffusing oils aromatically through the air stimulates smell receptors, which send signals to the part of the brain that governs emotional responses and regulates heart rate, blood pressure, stress levels, hormone balance, and memory. These oils can have potentially profound physiological and psychological effects.

Make a ritual out of acquainting yourself with one oil at a time. While scents like lavender and chamomile are widely given their due praise, there are many others that can bring their own calming properties into your space. The blends here feature essential oils known to promote relaxation and an easier transition into sleep as well as enhance the quality of sleep.

Before you begin, consider potency: one drop goes a long way. Blends are based on 100 ml of water and a suggested diffusing time of 30–60 minutes. Choose 100 percent pure organic or wildcrafted essential oils for your most therapeutic experience, adding drops to your diffuser and filling with water according to the user manual. Breathe in peace and breathe out relief.

PEACEFUL POTION: nightly soothing and healing vibes, inviting positive energy and creating ease inside:

★ 3 drops lavender

★ 3 drops bergamot

★ 2 drops vetiver

★ 1 drop sweet orange

★ 1 drop ylang ylang

SUNDOWN SERENADE: sedating and centering, bringing you back to a bedtime state of mind:

- ★ 2 drops neroli
- ★ 2 drops lavender
- ★ 2 drops frankincense
- ★ 1 drop lemon
- ★ 1 drop sandalwood
- ★ 1 drop patchouli

SWEET SANCTITY: enchanting and woodsy, reminiscent of a sacred mountain after an evening rain shower to help you sink into bliss:

- ★ 4 drops Palo Santo
- ★ 2 drops lemon balm
- ★ 2 drops black spruce
- ★ 2 drops cedarwood

MOON DUST: sacred release and invocation, helping you let go of everything but peace in the present moment:

- ★ 3 drops lavender
- ★ 2 drops sweet orange
- ★ 2 drops Palo Santo
- ★ 1 drop clary sage
- ★ 1 drop juniper berry
- ★ 1 drop cedarwood

HEART CONSTELLATIONS: alluring and mood-balancing, like a hypnotic chant of the sky and earth, calling you to sleep:

- ★ 3 drops sandalwood
- ★ 2 drops bergamot
- ★ 2 drops rose
- ★ 2 drops myrrh

STILL MOMENTS: down-to-earth yet uplifting, flowing like nectar to bless you with all the comfort of the universe:

- ★ 2 drops lavender
- ★ 2 drops bergamot
- ★ 2 drops sweet marjoram
- ★ 2 drops cypress
- ★ 1 drop lemon
- ★ 1 drop peppermint

MOONBEAM BLOSSOMS: ponder a celestial light shower watering your soul's beauty while you sleep:

- ★ 3 drops rose
- ★ 3 drops patchouli
- ★ 2 drops jasmine
- ★ 1 drop German chamomile
- ★ 1 drop ylang ylang

Cleansing and Elevating Your Space

3. COMFORTING VANILLA SIMMER

Simmering fresh and dried herbs, fruits, extracts, and spices on the stovetop is a heartwarming alternative to diffusing essential oils and safer than artificially-scented candles. The aromatic moisture that fills your space is an effective, easy, and pleasing way to bid the day farewell and greet the evening ahead.

Simmer pot recipes invoke the playful imagination—be as creative or simplistic as you want to be. Aside from fruits, consider fragrant ingredients like rosemary sprigs, rose petals, lavender flowers, fresh pine needles, bay leaves, juniper berries, cranberries, cinnamon sticks, clove buds, and anise. The recipes here use the lush, alluring aroma of vanilla (extract or spent vanilla bean pods) as a backdrop to melt away woes and attract blissful sleep.

Follow these instructions for each recipe:

1. Combine all ingredients in a cast iron pot, slow cooker, or a food-safe kitchen cauldron. For cleaning purposes, you may want to use a dedicated pot for simmering.
2. Add enough water to cover ingredients and bring to a boil. Turn down heat and simmer on low. Check on water level about once every 30 minutes and add water as needed. Do not let simmer pot burn dry.
3. Enjoy the warm, comforting scent wafting from your kitchen and blessing every room with positive earthy energy.

Use the following recipes as loose guidelines and then explore combinations to create your desired bedtime vibes with a little help from nature's bounty. For stronger scents, add more ingredients.

LUSCIOUS EARTH:

* 10 juniper berries (gently crush to release scent)
* 1 orange rind (add slices if desired)
* 2 cinnamon sticks
* 1 tablespoon whole cloves
* ½ teaspoon ground nutmeg
* 1 teaspoon almond extract
* 1 tablespoon vanilla extract or 1 vanilla bean pod

LAVENDER MAGIC:

* 2 tablespoons dried lavender flowers
* 2 tablespoons dried rose petals
* 5 whole star anise pods
* 1 tablespoon vanilla extract or 1 vanilla bean pod

TIME TO UNWIND:

* 1 apple peel (add slices if desired)
* 1 orange rind (add slices if desired)
* 1 lemon, sliced
* 2 cinnamon sticks
* 3–5 bay leaves
* ½ teaspoon ground nutmeg
* 1 tablespoon vanilla extract or 1 vanilla bean pod

One simmer pot recipe can be used for several days and composted once spent—treat this as an offering back to the earth. For premade recipes, place ingredients into a clean mason jar with water to designated fill line, cover, and refrigerate up to 1 week.

4. LULLABY LINEN MISTS

It is a comfort to go to bed with fresh sheets, but it is pure bliss when your sheets envelop you in the serene scents of lavender, chamomile, lemon balm, and bergamot. Surrounding yourself with certain aromas invites you into a relaxed mind-body state and can even positively influence your dreams once asleep. Lovingly craft your own blissful blends to cradle your deepest desires and support your deepest slumber. Offer aromatic blessings while you mist and visualize every molecule transforming your space into a haven for the weary soul.

To use these mists, combine ingredients into a 2-ounce misting bottle with a pinch of Epsom or sea salt. Add distilled water to fill bottle. Shake gently before each use. Mist liberally around your room and over your pillows, bed sheets, and body with intention and care for a soothing bedtime ritual. Lightly spritz dream pillows and herbal sleep sachets to refresh scents. If any of these mists resonate with your intentions for your whole home, you can incorporate them into your home blessing ceremonies.

Choose 100 percent pure organic or wildcrafted essential oils to make your favorite aromatherapy misters: use the sleep-inducing blends here to begin your journey into the night.

MOON MOODS: a grounding blend to balance the emotions and cradle the heart:

* ★ 4 drops sweet marjoram
* ★ 4 drops peppermint
* ★ 2 drops juniper berry
* ★ 2 drops cypress
* ★ ½ ounce lavender hydrosol

EVENING EMBRACE: an alluring blend to enchant and attract infinite possibilities:

- ★ 4 drops bergamot
- ★ 4 drops sandalwood
- ★ 2 drops jasmine
- ★ 2 drops ylang ylang
- ★ ½ ounce neroli hydrosol

HEAVENLY HAVEN: an earthy citrus blend to provide comfort and guidance:

- ★ 4 drops Palo Santo
- ★ 4 drops frankincense
- ★ 2 drops clary sage
- ★ 2 drops vetiver
- ★ ½ ounce lemon balm hydrosol

STAR DREAMS: a sedating blend to invite celestial wonder and grace:

- ★ 4 drops sweet orange
- ★ 4 drops patchouli
- ★ 4 drops cedarwood
- ★ ½ ounce rose hydrosol

PEACE ETERNAL: a sweet and herbaceous blend to release woes and warm the soul:

- ★ 4 drops bergamot
- ★ 4 drops lavender
- ★ 2 drops Roman chamomile
- ★ 2 drops rose
- ★ ½ ounce clary sage hydrosol

FRUITFUL SLUMBER: a soothing blend to encourage pleasant thoughts and sweet dreams:

- ★ 4 drops tangerine
- ★ 4 drops palmarosa
- ★ 4 drops clary sage
- ★ ½ ounce chamomile hydrosol

5. SAGE SMUDGING

Sage is a plant long revered for its ability to purify, protect, and elevate. In Native American tradition, the burning of sage, also known as smudging, is a sacred ritual of clearing stuck and unwanted energies from a person, thing, or space. Perform a smudging ceremony whenever your physical space and headspace could use an energetic lift—it could take just 10 minutes or less to totally relax. Cleansing negativity and welcoming in new positive energy provides a sense of safety and support as you prepare to sleep, helping you transition into a bedtime state of mind.

You will need:

★ A clear intention
★ A sage smudge stick
★ A wooden match
★ A heat-proof container (choose an abalone shell for additional purifying power)

Follow these steps with an attitude of reverence:

1. Open windows to allow for circulation of fresh air.
2. Speak your intention for purification and mentally recite throughout the ceremony. Ask that all emotions and energies that do not resonate with your intention be removed: try something like "I release all energies that do not serve me" or "May this space be filled with peace."
3. Light sage with a wooden match. Wait about 30 seconds, then blow out flame and let stick smolder. Fan embers lightly to keep smoldering (may need to be re-lit). Use a shell, pottery, or other non-flammable container to catch ashes.

4. Allow smoke to billow around you, working your way up from your feet to your head and back down. Visualize your spirit being cleansed, absolving all negativity.

5. Moving in a clockwise direction, beginning from the east, lightly wave sage stick around your home. Use your hand or a feather to waft smoke in all directions. Pay attention to high-traffic areas, windows, doorways, floorboards, closets, corners, and any sacred ritual tools (crystals, dream catchers) that need cleansing. Imagine the smoke carrying your intention or prayer into every nook and cranny.

6. When done, extinguish sage stick by pressing it gently against the inside of your container. Store in a dry, dark place, out of reach of children and animals.

OTHER HERBS

Sage smudge sticks sometimes come bundled with other herbs. You can add any of the following herbs to give your cleansing ritual an energetic boost:

★ Lavender: Peace. Healing. Relaxation. Restful sleep.
★ Frankincense: Connection with spirit. Reduce stress. Ease tension.
★ Thyme: Release the past. Healing.
★ Chamomile: Protection. Purification.
★ Rosemary: Spiritual healing. Youth. Purification of energy associated with sickness. Ward off nightmares. Emotional support.
★ Cloves: Comfort for the bereaved. Protection.
★ Roses: Attract love and domestic peace.

6. BURNING PALO SANTO

Sourced from fallen branches of the fragrant mystical tree, the scent of smoldering Palo Santo sticks is at once uplifting and grounding. Sweet notes of mint and citrus lend a heavenly presence while its light woodsy smoke offers gifts of purification and good fortune. (Fittingly, its name means "holy wood" in Spanish.) Long revered for its constellation of medicinal and therapeutic properties, Palo Santo is traditionally used to relieve headaches, inflammation, cold and flu symptoms, and emotional trauma—removing obstacles to a peaceful slumber. Invoke the spiritually healing qualities of its smoke come evening to clear negative energy, strengthen vitality, bestow divine blessings, and pave the way for an effortless night's sleep.

You will need:

* 1 wild-harvested, ethically sourced Palo Santo stick (often sold in bundles)
* A match or candle
* An abalone shell or fireproof bowl of metal, glass, or clay

As you move through this sacred plant ceremony, expect a pleasant and refreshing experience, like a nature walk after a rainstorm:

1. Use a candle or match to light your Palo Santo stick. Hold over fireproof bowl or shell while it burns for about 30 seconds. Gently blow out flame. Blow on embers to keep smoke going throughout the process and relight as many times as needed.

2. Offer up a silent prayer, such as "I ask that the spirit of Palo Santo graciously fill this space with blessings."

3. Begin at the front door and mindfully move through your space in a clockwise direction. Allow the healing smoke to fill the room, wafting with your hand or a feather to assist.

4. Thank the rising smoke for lifting away misfortune and negative thoughts while simultaneously raising the energetic vibrations of your space, any tools you use for rituals, and yourself. Feel yourself cleansed of stress.

5. When your ritual is complete, place your Palo Santo stick in its fireproof container. The flame will eventually go out on its own. Keep out of reach of children, animals, and flammable materials.

FOR SMOKELESS CLEANSING

Though usually lit for ceremonial purposes, Palo Santo is fragrant in its raw form and doesn't necessarily need to be lit to enjoy a peaceful ambience before bed. For smokeless cleansing, you can:

★ Place sticks on your nightstand, altar, or in safe locations around the home.

★ Diffuse drops of Palo Santo essential oil with its botanical cousin, frankincense, and citrus oils to protect, purify, and enlighten.

★ Place a drop of Palo Santo essential oil in the palm of your hand, gently rub palms together, and bring them to your face as you inhale its rich fragrance.

7. DREAMCATCHER CEREMONY

The dreamcatcher is a spiritual object and part of a cherished tradition originating from Native American culture. Legend involves a teacher of wisdom appearing as a spider who wove a web of feathers, beads, and other natural elements to sift dreams, visions, and vibrations for its sleeping people. As the web catches bad dreams and unwanted energies, good dreams are allowed to pass through the center hole. Any lingering negativity is burned away in the morning light. The dreamcatcher is believed to provide spiritual protection and bring you into harmony with your deepest desires while you sleep.

Blessing your dreamcatcher is a customary way to pay respect and ensure that it works for you. Use this ceremony for initiation and cleansing to support your journey into a restful slumber:

1. Choose an open space or window to hang your dreamcatcher.
2. Open windows to allow fresh air to circulate and assist the cleansing process.
3. Place crystals near or underneath the dreamcatcher. Clear quartz, smoky quartz, and black tourmaline work well in this ritual.
4. When ready, stand in the center of the room and light a white sage bundle, Palo Santo, or incense. Holding over a shell or fireproof container, let the smoke purify you first as you waft it around the perimeter of your body.
5. Offer prayers for purification and protection as you waft smoke in all four directions—North, East, South, West. Offer to the sky and the boundless wisdom of the universe.

Offer to the ground, thanking Mother Earth for her endless support and nurturance.

6. Next, lightly waft smoke around the dreamcatcher, beginning at the front.

7. Speak out loud to your dreamcatcher as a friend and an extension of yourself. Voice your intentions and visualize these desires being woven into its web. Thank it for watching over you and for the goodness it will perform.

8. When finished, let smoke burn out or press gently to extinguish in the container.

9. Meditate on the feeling of the weight being lifted from the air and walls. Believe in the energetic power of your dreamcatcher, ready to guide you safely to Dreamland.

While the materials are laced with symbolism, what gives the dreamcatcher its power is your devoted intention. Handle with care and mend any loose threads. Do not wash with water. Periodically set out in the moonlight or morning light for an hour or so for additional purification.

SMOKELESS CLEANSING

For a smokeless ceremony, use a smudging mist. In a 2-ounce spray bottle, combine the following ingredients and shake gently before lightly misting around your dreamcatcher:

★ ½ ounce chamomile hydrosol
★ 12 drops essential oils: 4 drops clary sage, 4 drops lemon, 4 drops lavender
★ Distilled water to fill

8. FOUR CORNERS HOME PROTECTION

Sea salt is as versatile in sacred rituals as it is in the kitchen. When it comes to guarding your home against negative vibes and nightmares, humble salt might not seem powerful enough, but ancient traditions (that are still alive today) say otherwise. Some of salt's supposed spiritual properties include cleansing, purification, grounding, and protection—making this kitchen staple a viable smoke-free alternative to cleansing your space of unrestful energy. A strong intention, of course, is what sparks the transformation. With it, you can do something as simple as keeping a bowl of salt in the four corners of your home to feel more balanced, positive, and prepared for a restful sleep.

You will need:

★ An intention for purification and protection

★ 4 glass vessels

★ 2 teaspoons sea salt (white, pink, or black), divided

★ Essential oils of clary sage, lemon, and Palo Santo

★ ¼ teaspoon white sage leaves (optional)

★ Filtered or spring water

Prepare and perform this salt ritual with your intention in the front of your mind.

1. In each of your glass vessels, combine: 2 drops each clary sage, lemon, and Palo Santo essential oils; ½ teaspoon sea salt; and a pinch of sage leaves if using.

2. Stir ingredients to distribute scent and purifying properties. Fill about halfway with filtered or spring water and stir again.

3. Over each of your vessels, speak or silently recite your intention for purification and protection. Imagine your

intentions being programmed into the water. You can choose something simple, such as "Please absorb all negativity and unrest from this home, leaving me (us) free to sleep in peace."

4. Locate the four corners of your home. You can use a free compass app to familiarize yourself with the directions of your space.

5. Move in a clockwise direction and place each vessel in the four corners of your home—North, East, South, and West. Envision with each placement that a grid is being created, sealing off and protecting the energy of your space.

6. When you are finished, stand in the center of your home and once again speak or silently recite your intention. Thank the natural substances of the earth for actively absorbing all negative and unrestful energy while you sleep.

7. Empty the vessels as part of tomorrow evening's ritual sequence, simply pouring contents into the ground as an offering back to the earth, which will receive the natural materials and recycle them into new neutral energy.

8. Repeat as often as necessary, beginning with fresh ingredients each night, until you feel as though your space is cleansed and supportive of peaceful sleep.

To make your ritual feel even more powerful, incorporate sound healing tools such as chanting, clapping, bells, drums, or singing bowls.

9. CRYSTAL GRIDDING

Creating a crystal grid is a way to organize the energetic power of crystals using the concept of sacred geometry, the "language" of the universe. The purpose is to enhance a specific intention, such as clearing mental space, healing today's hurts, and peaceful sleep. By arranging choice crystals into symmetrical patterns, you are conspiring with the universe to manifest your desires. You don't need expertise to restructure the energy of your space—the "magic" is in your intention.

Use the crystals you already have and any other natural materials (such as petals, leaves, sticks, and feathers) to craft a visual reminder of your intention for peace, healing, or comfort tonight. The following instructions provide a basic template to work from:

1. Dedicate a safe place away from other hands and paws—a special room, corner, or altar.

2. Cleanse your space and crystals if needed using sacred smoke, sound clearing, or a blessing.

3. Choose a larger center stone for the focal point of the grid. Though not necessary, a pointed clear quartz crystal is effective at transmitting energy.

4. Write down a single, clear intention on a piece of paper and place underneath your center stone. "I wish for peaceful sleep" or "I am willing to release today" are examples.

5. Choose up to three additional crystal types to surround the center crystal. Let your intuition guide you in any symmetrical placement, forming at least three "layers" of crystals.

6. Now it is time to "activate" your grid. Choose a natural cut stone that's at least 2 inches long with a tapered end as your activation wand.

7. Point the wand at the center stone and visualize universal energy beaming through you, into the wand. Slowly move the wand from stone to stone, connecting the dots, directing your intentions and energy into each stone.

8. Once all stones are "activated," visualize your intention coming to fruition and aligning with the greatest good of all beings. Close your eyes and breathe in this reality.

Your grid can be as small as a coaster or as large as a room. To easily grid a room, add four clear quartz points in each corner facing inward. Leave your grid up for a week, until the next moon, or until finished with a meditation practice.

MATCHING CRYSTALS TO INTENTION

There are as many intentions as there are stars in the sky. Luckily, each crystal has a unique energy vibration to support your deepest desires. Here are some to consider as you journey into peaceful sleep:

★ Love: Rose quartz; Rhodonite; Chrysoprase
★ Hope and healing: Rainbow obsidian; Blue lace agate; Amazonite
★ Good dreams: Celestite; Labradorite; Smoky quartz
★ Peace of mind: Amethyst; Lepidolite; Sodalite

10. COMMUNING WITH PLANT CONSCIOUSNESS

Your intentional connection with the natural world is incredibly calming. Thus, one of the best ways to design a peaceful sleep environment is to bring nature indoors. This relaxing ritual embraces the idea that plants are sentient beings with personalities, feelings, and unique energy. Borrowing techniques from ancient shamanic traditions of communicating with plant spirits, this is simply an opportunity to appreciate the natural offerings of Mother Earth. It might just mean that you spend a little more time respectfully tending to your house plants, especially those that promote healthy sleep patterns.

Follow these steps to deepen your plant relationships and your sleep:

1. Open your heart to believing that you can commune with plant consciousness. Relax into a childlike curiosity. Let your imagination lead the way. Set an intention to connect, such as "I am open to the healing energy of plants."

2. Approach each plant, one at a time, with genuine respect and a feeling of awe and appreciation. Notice its colors, scents, number of petals, and formation of leaves. Spend time examining with your five senses.

3. Talk to the plant in a caring tone—you can commune silently, knowing that plants respond to your feelings. Compliment its health and progress, and note that as it grows and flourishes, so do you.

4. Touch the plant and close your eyes as you focus on caressing the plant with your fingertips. Imagine your consciousness merging with the plant's.

5. Take your awareness inward and notice how you feel around this plant. Be aware of your breathing. Notice how plants are always meditating, surrendering in the flow of life. Notice any sensations or impressions that appear in your mind's eye, even if you do not understand them.

6. When you are ready to move on to the next plant, thank this plant for purifying and infusing your home with restful energy. Leave an offering: a blessing, some water, a trimming if needed, repositioning, or simply your respectful awareness.

7. Continue until you have moved through all of your plants or feel you are finished. Stay with the collective plant consciousness for one last moment, honoring its help creating a healing space while you sleep.

SLEEP-FRIENDLY PLANTS

Consider bringing these plants and flowers into your bedroom and home for their uplifting, cleansing, and calming qualities:

★ Rosemary: Spiritual healing. Stress relief. Air purification. Ward off nightmares.

★ Sage: Sedative. General well-being.

★ Lavender, Chamomile: Reduce anxiety. Lift mood. Deepen sleep. Relaxation.

★ Jasmine: Reduce anxiety. Emotional balance. Soothe mind and body.

★ Valerian, Gardenia: Improve sleep quality. Ease insomnia.

★ English Ivy, Spider Plant, Snake Plant, Peace Lily, Aloe Vera: Improve air quality at night for easy breathing.

11. MAGIC MOON DANCE

Similar to how rainmaking ceremonies are performed to invoke the resource and blessing of water, this manifestation ritual pays reverence to the moon with your entire body in exchange for the offering of healing sleep. As you bring slow, fluid movements into the body, you lubricate the joints, corral a wandering mind, and fill your space with positive energy. Your intuitive approach to this dance sparks an intimate connection with the rhythms of nature—the moon and her tides, your body and its sleep cycles—and leaves you feeling harmonized, calm, and in control of your environment. In other words, you assume the energetic qualities of the moon; sleeping easy is only natural.

This is a potent ritual *because* it is deeply personal. Use the following steps as a loose guideline as you practice moving in ways that honor your body, space, and sleep. There is no wrong way to dance with the moon:

1. Choose a space with enough room to move about— indoors or outdoors (though indoors brings energy directly into your space). Incorporate any elements that symbolize the moon or evoke peace: crystals (moonstone, opal, labradorite), fairy lights, shamanic music.

2. Feet rooted in the earth, speak a sleep-focused intention: "May my space and I be renewed by the healing light of the moon."

3. Open your arms wide to embrace the moon. Visualize breathing in moonlight through the crown of your head and heart, sending sustenance to every cell with your exhale.

4. Come into a slow dance that feels good, effortless, and liberating. Allow your creative energy to arise within you and direct your movement. Dance to commune with the moon.

5. Explore all directions—high, low, side to side, diagonal, turning—oscillating and undulating. Be respectful of your knees, neck, and low back. Every movement is a rhythmic massage. Enjoy the spontaneous unfolding.

6. Meander through your space without restraint or judgment. Flow as though you were swimming. Be light on your feet.

7. Sense the moon and the movement dislodging tensions and fear inside—freeing you from whatever binds you. Dance in a field of infinite possibilities and cellular intelligence.

8. Sense internal spaciousness growing. Allow your whole body to receive the infinite blessings of the moon: peace, sleep, renewal. Surrender to the flow. Rest in the support.

9. With care, come back to center.

10. Inhale and sweep your arms up toward the sky. Exhale and, palms together, bring your hands down in front of you. Repeat. Radiant drops of peaceful moon energy pour through you, spreading through your space. Inhale sustenance. Exhale respect.

11. With palms together in front of your heart, thank the moon for lending its energy, dancing with you, and making a reciprocal offering of sleep.

12. PEACEFUL HOME BLESSING

Home blessings are well known for activating space with positive intention. With endless possibilities for intentions, this ritual focuses on infusing the home with the blessing of peaceful sleep. Since your living space reflects and affects your internal space, the idea is that as you bless your home with serenity, you also bless yourself.

You will need:

* A heartfelt blessing
* A candle
* A devotional offering of your choosing: crystals, fresh flowers, dried herbs, white rice
* Many Blessings Spray (see following recipe) (optional)
* A sound healing tool: singing bowl, bell, chime, etc. (optional)

For your blessing, choose the phrasing that feels right for your current sleep patterns and state of mind. For example: "May this home be a restful haven for the mind, body, and soul. May I be comforted by the peace held within these walls. May sleep come easily tonight and life be new tomorrow. And so it is." A simple "Bless this home with the energy of sleep" also works.

To activate your home with your blessing:

1. Begin in an open living space where you can safely light a candle to burn while you walk through your home.
2. Light your candle with the intention of welcoming in blessings.
3. Speak or silently recite your blessing as you walk around the perimeter of your home. If you are using the Many Blessings

Spray, you can mist while you walk, imagining every molecule infusing blessings into your space.

4. Each time you reach a corner, speak or think: "And so it is." If you are using a sound healing tool (such as a bell or chime), you can include that here to seal the blessing.

5. As a gesture of gratitude, leave a devotional offering of your choosing wherever you feel called to: on windowsills, tables, in the center of each room, on an altar, etc. Put fresh flowers in a vase for beautiful dreams. Leave a sprig of dried herbs, like lavender for peace. Leave an amethyst crystal for healing sleep. Sprinkle white rice on windowsills for abundant support.

6. When you have made your way back to your candle, extinguish the flame with care. Envision the smoke carrying your blessings higher to be answered and supported by the entire universe.

A home blessing ritual is especially powerful when done after a sacred home cleansing ritual (such as smudging).

MANY BLESSINGS SPRAY

Combine the following ingredients in a 2-ounce spray bottle with water to welcome the qualities of love, peace, and joy into your sleep space:

- ★ 4 drops sandalwood essential oil
- ★ 4 drops jasmine essential oil
- ★ 4 drops neroli essential oil
- ★ ½ ounce rose hydrosol

CHAPTER 3

CLEANSING AND PREPARING YOUR BODY

Regular therapeutic touch opens the floodgates for healing: it reduces pain, improves mood, calms symptoms of depression and anxiety, and improves sleep quality, thanks to its release of the neurotransmitter serotonin. You don't even need another pair of hands to introduce healing vibrations into your night. However you apply your loving touch, the decision to do so communicates that you value sleep, the ultimate gift of restoration.

The rituals in this chapter are about valuing your sleep by valuing your body. Your body is always showing up for you, listening and responding to you, doing its best to give you a full experience of life. Approaching your body with that same level of commitment is a radical act of self-care and one that can revolutionize your sleep.

Each ritual is a treat and a peace treaty. You're practicing giving yourself permission to receive the graces of an open heart and an opportunity to heal. Follow these two steps with any ceremony you feel called to apply tonight:

★ Take a moment to notice the parts of your body that need loving attention. No need to avoid whatever shows up. No need to suppress negative voices. Only feel the need to be there with a curious and compassionate willingness to see, to hear, to learn.

★ Answer needs with a generous solution: ritual instead of reprimand. Cleanse with reverence. Know that you are inviting new rhythms, promoting what you love, and tasting the kind of nourishment sleep gives so naturally and generously.

Something that takes just 5 minutes to do can change the way you interpret your day, the way you understand yourself, and the way you feel when you wake up tomorrow.

1. DRY BRUSHING

This ancient Ayurvedic technique is an easy and inexpensive way to thank your body at the end of the day. Brushing your skin is a natural exfoliating and detoxifying process, as it unclogs pores and stimulates the lymphatic system, promoting the flow of oxygen and nutrients and the removal of impurities. Since your skin is full of touch receptors, dry brushing is a comforting treat for the nervous system and a powerful way to calm frazzled nerves before bed. Light a candle as an additional reminder that all is well and you are safe tonight.

For a heart-opening experience, worship yourself with loving attention. Be mindful of each stroke on your skin, brushing stress and worries away with the toxins and dead cells. This is a time to allow your mind to quiet and your body to breathe. Your ritual can take as little as a few minutes and as long as twenty; just be sure to go slowly and meditatively.

Perform this ritual prior to your nightly bath when your skin is completely dry—about 2 hours before bed. Follow the following steps for polished and peaceful results:

1. Select a dry brush (you can find them online or in health stores) with natural bristles and a long handle for hard-to-reach places.

2. Stand in the shower or on a towel to catch any dead skin that falls off.

3. Always brush toward the heart with light pressure, and brush each area of your body several times (work your way up to ten times) before moving on to the next area. If uncomfortable, use less pressure.

4. Start with the soles of your feet in a circular motion. Move up your legs with long, smooth, sweeping strokes.

5. Repeat this process with the palms of your hands, moving up your arms toward your heart.

6. Continue with your buttocks and back, brushing upward, followed by the back of your neck, brushing down.

7. Finish with your stomach, armpits, and chest, brushing with even lighter pressure in a circular clockwise motion.

8. If you decide to brush your face, use a separate, smaller, softer brush designed for this purpose. Begin with clean skin, brushing in a circular motion all over before brushing down your T-zone and down your cheeks, finishing with long strokes from chin to chest. Perform two or three times a week.

You may choose to finish with a moisturizing oil like organic coconut or jojoba. Wash your brush once a week or every two weeks with mild soap and warm water, placing bristle side down in a sunny spot to dry.

Notes: Medium pressure is about as intense as you want to get. Your skin will become less sensitive the more you dry brush. Skin may be slightly pink afterward, but it should not be red or painful. Avoid cuts or rashes. You may want to skip this practice if you have extremely sensitive skin or bothersome skin conditions.

2. LUXURIOUS MILK AND SALT BATH

Immersion in water is therapeutic on its own, helping you detach from the hyper-connectedness of the modern world. This warm ritual bath elevates the experience into something special with mineral-rich salts, nourishing milk, anti-inflammatory and antioxidant oats, relaxing plant essences, and your own sacred awareness. The thoughtful blend of functional ingredients produces a calming aromatic atmosphere for mind, body, and soul. It soothes sore muscles, removes physical and energetic impurities, replenishes magnesium levels, melts away stress, and cues a cooling-down period afterward—all important for a blissful night's sleep, night after night.

You will need:

- ★ 2 cups drinking water
- ★ Desired elements to enhance space: salt lamp, candles, crystals, music, book, journal
- ★ Medium mixing bowl
- ★ 2 tablespoons ground oats
- ★ 2 tablespoons dried herbs of choice: lavender flowers, rose petals, chamomile flowers, hibiscus flowers
- ★ ¼ cup Epsom salt
- ★ ¼ cup Himalayan salt or sea salt
- ★ 5–10 drops essential oils of choice: lavender, rose, neroli, peppermint
- ★ Large reusable or disposable tea filter of choice: cloth, paper, organza, or muslin bag
- ★ 1 cup full-fat milk: cow, goat, coconut

When you need a little extra help loosening up and calming down, treat yourself to this cleansing, balancing bath an hour and a half before bedtime.

Instructions:

1. Mindfully create a sacred space using desired elements from the previous list. While preparing, drink 1 cup of water to hydrate.

2. Combine ingredients in a mixing bowl: oats through essential oils.

3. Scoop mixture into filter. Tie drawstrings or staple for a tight seal.

4. Add filter to running bath water and swirl or gently squeeze to dissolve.

5. Add milk just before stepping in.

6. Slowly enter the water as if you are entering a healing pool of rejuvenation. Offer a blessing, such as "I cleanse myself of stress. I bathe in peace."

7. While soaking (20–30 minutes), imagine the water removing anything you came to release, replenishing you with what you need for a peaceful sleep. Enjoy your time here.

8. End with gratitude for the beauty you created before draining every last bit of energetic debris from today. Optionally you can rinse with a shower. Throw the filter (or just its contents) away.

9. Drink the second cup of water to rehydrate.

PREMADE BATH RECIPE

Once you have a scent you love, use this make-ahead recipe, good for four to eight baths. Combine all ingredients in a mixing bowl and stir until well distributed. Store in airtight glass jars. Add 1 cup mixture in filter(s) to running bath water.

★ 2 cups powdered milk: cow, goat, coconut
★ 1 cup ground oats
★ 1 cup dried herbs
★ 2 cups Epsom salt
★ 2 cups Himalayan salt or sea salt
★ 40–80 drops essential oils

3. COOLING SHOWER

Cooling down is a signal that sleep is near. Though taking a warm bath 90 minutes before bed is a relaxing way to end the day, starting too close to bedtime can interrupt the body's natural cooling down process. On those later nights, especially after a day of strenuous activity and heat, a cooling shower ritual might be just what your tired body needs. Cold-water hydrotherapy touts anti-depressant and anti-inflammatory effects, improves circulation and immunity, and speeds recovery of hardworking muscles. In Kundalini yoga tradition, a cool shower is believed to help the body self-regulate and ready itself for a healing night of deep, uninterrupted sleep.

Here are some ways to gradually turn a cooling shower into a therapeutic evening ritual—maybe even a treat that you look forward to:

★ Splash cold water on your feet, wrists, face, and armpits if you're not ready for a whole-body immersion.

★ End your normal bath or shower with 15 seconds of cooler water. Gradually progress to a minute, working your way up to about 3 minutes.

★ Visualize the cool water cascading down as if you were standing underneath a waterfall on a warm, sunny summer's day. Imagine yourself bathing in warm light while this waterfall pours over you. Immerse yourself in that experience.

★ Focus on your purification. Concentrate on how wonderful it feels to be standing under this refreshing water as it falls and washes away all stress, clears all debris, and sends every bit of lingering unwanted energy down the drain.

★ Visualize your joints and muscles being nourished as inflammation subsides and toxins are released. This is your way of thanking your body for doing its best today.

★ Practice gratitude for the life-giving miracle of clean water. While you're at it, you may want to mentally scroll through other gifts, such as shelter and breath and the opportunity to practice something solely because it's good for you.

★ Repeat a healing affirmation or mantra that reflects how you are helping yourself and how you want to feel, such as "I am taking care of myself" or "I love my body and my body loves me."

★ Add a few drops of relaxing or mood-lifting essential oils to a washcloth and place on the shower floor for an aromatic experience. Try lavender, clary sage, bergamot, sweet marjoram, Roman chamomile, vetiver, ylang ylang, or another personal favorite.

When you are finished, thank yourself with a Self-Loving Oil Massage (see ritual in this chapter). Settle into a bed that feels a little cozier than usual—with fresh sheets, a clean body, and a clear mind that's receptive to sleep.

4. EPSOM SALT FOOT SOAK

If sinking into the tub is simply not going to happen tonight, soaking your feet in Epsom salt is a simple treat and an efficient way to absorb magnesium—an essential mineral that soothes the nervous system and supports several bodily functions. Stress, caffeine, alcohol, refined sugar, and prescription medications deplete magnesium reserves, leading to muscle spasms and cramps, chronic pain, and difficulty falling and staying asleep. A magnesium-rich foot soak serves as necessary replenishment for the entire body. Featuring calming herbs and comforting oils, this recipe helps reduce pain and inflammation, steadies internal rhythms, and aids the immune system. You will be left feeling smooth and pampered—inside and out.

In Chinese medicine, salt assists the downward flow of energy, making a foot soak especially beneficial at the end of a busy day. Soak about one hour before bedtime to feel grounded, calm, and connected to your body.

You will need:

★ Desired elements to enhance space: candles, music, book

★ A large basin or pot, to soak both feet

★ Warm to hot water to fill basin (a tolerable temperature that won't cool too quickly or burn)

★ ¼ cup Epsom salts

★ 1 tablespoon carrier oil of choice: jojoba, sesame, olive, sweet almond, rose

★ 3–4 drops essential oils of choice: lavender and peppermint, rosemary, cedarwood and rose

★ 1 tablespoon each, dried: lavender flowers, chamomile flowers, rose petals

★ Additional body oil for a
  lower leg massage (can be
  the same as your carrier oil)

★ A towel

Instructions:

1. Choose a comfortable place to do your foot soak: light a few
   candles; play soft music; have a book nearby.

2. Pour warm to hot water into your basin.

3. Sprinkle Epsom salt, carrier oil, essential oils, and flowers
   into the water and stir until completely dissolved.

4. Soak your feet in the mixture 15–30 minutes, or until water
   cools. While soaking, massage body oil into your ankles, calves,
   and knees. Pay attention to the inside of your lower legs.

5. When finished, remove feet from water and pat dry with a
   towel. Apply body oil to lock in moisture or follow with a
   Magnesium Oil Foot Massage (see this chapter). Perform
   once or twice a week, or as often as needed.

PREMADE FOOT SOAK

Refer to the following ingredients for a make-ahead recipe,
good for four foot soaks. In a large bowl, mix carrier oil and
essential oils. Add Epsom salt and herbs until mixed well.
Store in an airtight glass container in a cool, dry place.

★ 4 tablespoons carrier oil

★ 12–16 drops essential oils of choice

★ 2 cups Epsom salt

★ 4 tablespoons each, dried: lavender flowers, chamomile
  flowers, rose petals

5. NURTURING SUGAR SCRUB

Soothing for hard-working hands and gentle enough for the face, this nighttime sugar scrub ritual communicates self-love and appreciation. While exfoliation is considered an essential element of skincare for its beautifying benefits—encouraging cell turnover and smooth, glowing skin—it can be a deeply nourishing experience mentally and emotionally. By taking your time, you are unwinding tangled thoughts and intentionally feeling for the pulse of the present moment. The true gift is in the beauty sleep that follows this kind of loving attention.

Try the following and slow down as you soften your skin, muscles, heart, and perspective:

1. With clean hands, prepare your sugar scrub (see recipe that follows). Over a sink, scoop about 1 teaspoon of the scrub with a clean spoon, taking care not to get water in the container.

2. With extraordinarily gentle circular motions, massage the muscles of your face—jaw, cheeks, nose, temples, forehead—for about 3 minutes. Be mindful of the texture against your skin and the relaxing scent.

3. Rinse with warm water and then cool water before patting the skin dry with a soft towel.

4. Massage your favorite serum, lotion, or oil in the same loving manner to lock in moisture: jojoba, argan, avocado, coconut, or rose hip seed oil is beneficial depending on skin type.

5. Repeat this process as you scrub one elbow at a time in circular motions for about 1 minute each.

6. Moving down your forearms in longer strokes, consciously caress one hand at a time for about 3 minutes

each—wrists, palms, fingers, the tops of the hands. Breathe deeply as tension is extracted.

7. Rinse, pat dry, lock in moisture, and sigh with gratitude.

Use this sugar scrub recipe one to three times per week on the face, elbows, and hands. For a little more love, apply to the knees, feet, and entire body in the tub before showering (use extra caution, as the oil can make your tub slippery). Test on a small portion of skin and stop using immediately if the skin reacts; avoid broken or irritated skin.

You will need:

★ 1 cup organic brown sugar
★ ½ cup oil of choice: olive, coconut, apricot, sweet almond
★ ½ teaspoon vitamin E oil
★ 2 tablespoons raw honey (optional)
★ 10–20 drops of essential oils of choice: lavender, neroli, rose (optional)
★ 1 tablespoon dried flowers of choice: lavender flowers, rose petals (optional)
★ Airtight glass container(s)

Instructions:

1. Blend sugar, oil, vitamin E oil, and honey (if using) in a small mixing bowl.
2. Add essential oils if using and mix again.
3. If you'd like, gently fold in dried flowers.
4. Store in airtight glass containers in a cool, dry place. Use within 1 month.

Tip: For a face mask, use enough oil to make a thick paste. Slather on your face and leave on for 10–20 minutes before rinsing.

6. HERBAL FACIAL STEAM

A good old-fashioned steam is a blissful experience sure to encourage relaxation and the release of any lingering impurities from the day. This timeless self-care remedy is used to open pores, soften and hydrate skin, improve circulation, and unclog sinuses for easier breathing and sleeping. A steaming session prompts the steady decline in body temperature post-steam, encouraging the release of melatonin. Bring in beneficial aromatic herbs and feel the stress melt away.

Create a spa-like atmosphere for ultimate indulgence: choose a favorite space, dim the lights, light a candle, plug in the fairy lights, grace your eardrums with beautiful music, and adorn your body in a beautiful garment or your favorite pajamas. With everything around you emitting a soothing warmth, your pampering self-care ritual can begin. Enjoy this steam once or twice weekly.

You will need:

- ★ Tea kettle
- ★ Large heat-safe bowl and a lid
- ★ Small mixing bowl
- ★ 2 hand towels
- ★ ¼ cup dried herbal blend (see following suggestions)

Instructions:

1. Fill your kettle with water and heat until boiling.
2. While waiting for water to boil, gently mix your herbs in a small bowl. Fold one towel in half and place on a flat surface. Place your large heat-safe bowl on top of the towel.
3. Once boiling, carefully pour water into your heat-safe bowl.

4. Sprinkle herbs into the water, stirring and covering with lid for 1–2 minutes to steep.

5. Drape the other towel over the back of your head as you lean forward over bowl, creating a steam tent with your face at least 6 inches away to ensure a tolerable temperature.

6. Breathe slowly through your nose as you absorb the aromatic goodness. Bask in your own personal cocoon-like sanctuary for about 10 minutes or finish when the water is no longer giving off steam, or whenever you are ready.

7. Follow by rinsing your face with cool water to close your pores and pat dry. Massage your favorite natural oil or serum into your skin with love. Pour water outside somewhere safe as an offering back to the earth.

HERBAL BLENDS

Make your own apothecary blend using organic or wild-crafted and sustainably sourced ingredients based on your specific preferences or needs. Begin your exploration with a delicate blend of:

★ 2 parts each rose petals, chamomile flowers, and calendula flowers

★ 1 part each lavender flowers, yarrow leaf and flower, and white willow bark

Use ¼ cup per facial steam, store remaining ingredients in an airtight glass container out of direct sunlight—optionally add a citrus peel before each use.

7. MAGNESIUM OIL FOOT MASSAGE

With over 7,000 nerve endings and various meridian points clustered in each foot, giving both a massage before bed helps loosen the entire body. You may be delighted to discover how nightly sessions can support your overall well-being—from your mental and emotional health to the quality of your sleep. By stimulating the lymphatic system and the release of anti-pain chemicals, you can enjoy improved blood flow, lower blood pressure, and relief from a variety of ailments, including restless leg syndrome, edema, headaches, migraines, backaches, neck pain, premenstrual syndrome, menopause, depression, anxiety, insomnia, general stress, and fatigue. A little self-care really does go a long way.

Give yourself this grounding and uplifting gift whenever you need an extra touch of grace in your life:

1. Sit comfortably with one clean foot in your lap.
2. Rub oil into your hands or spray directly onto the foot (see following recipe). Apply more as needed throughout the massage.
3. Apply light relaxing strokes to the entire foot. Squeeze or knead—whatever feels good.
4. Press your thumb lightly into the base of your shin and drag toward your big toe. Repeat for each toe.
5. Press your thumb into and all around the pad of your big toe.
6. Gently squeeze and twist one toe at a time, from root to top, ending with the little toe.
7. Apply firmer thumb pressure along the ball of the foot, using big circles from the little toe to the big toe. Squeeze with your hand if that is more comfortable.

8. Apply light thumb pressure along the inner border of the sole, using small circles from the big toe to the heel.

9. Massage all around the heels and ankles with both hands. Gently squeeze around the Achilles tendon.

10. Inhale, pressing into the center of the heel for a few seconds. Exhale and release.

11. Apply light thumb pressure along the outer border of the sole, using small circles from the heel to the little toe.

12. Make a fist and knead the sole in small circles.

13. Locate the Solar Plexus point: squeeze both sides of your foot together to find the hollow that forms. Inhale and apply firm thumb pressure here for a few seconds. Exhale and release.

14. Finish with long relaxing strokes to the entire foot.

15. Repeat on the other foot.

16. Rinse or wipe down once absorbed and apply a moisturizer.

OIL FOR FOOT RUBS

The magnesium and essential oils in this recipe deliver stress-relieving properties to encourage your best sleep:

1. In a 4-ounce squeeze or spray bottle, combine almost 4 ounces magnesium oil with 10–20 drops each lavender and frankincense essential oil or another favorite combination such as: cedarwood and vetiver, or peppermint and sweet marjoram.

2. Shake gently to mix before each use. You may experience a tingling sensation at first; this should subside with regular use. Do not use on burns, open or healing wounds, fractures, or severe osteoporosis.

8. SELF-LOVING OIL MASSAGE

Your physical presence on earth is worthy of celebration—pay homage with your own therapeutic touch. A self-massage stimulates the release of endorphins, which not only makes you feel loved but reduces pain, enhances immune function, calms the nervous system, and promotes sound sleep. Through the application of oil plus kindness, you design a nurturing environment that turns off your inner critic and activates your innate healing power. In the space that's created, a sense of stability, warmth, and comfort can sink in.

Practice this evening sequence for a totally transformative experience—let your touch be slow, gentle, and firm; let your awareness be one of gratitude and respect:

1. Put your chosen oil blend in a squeeze or pump bottle for easy application. Warm oil in a container or sink filled with warm water. Roll bottle between palms to re-blend.

2. Undress and stand or sit on a designated towel or mat that can get oily. Keep a warm towel fresh from the dryer nearby to pat dry, if needed.

3. Rub a small amount of oil between your palms and massage your scalp with your fingertips in a circular motion. If you don't want oil in your hair, omit oil here.

4. Continue with your temples, face, ears, and nape of the neck in slow, circular movements. Massage your throat in upward movements. If using essential oils, avoid eyes and mucous membranes or omit oil here.

5. Continue with your arms and legs in the direction of your heart, applying even pressure with long strokes on muscles and circular movements on joints.

6. Massage your chest and abdomen with light pressure in a clockwise direction.

7. Move to your hips and bottom before paying attention to the soles of your feet and palms of each hand.

8. Allow oil to absorb for 5–20 minutes before bathing or leave oil on overnight, optionally using cotton socks and gloves to lock in moisture.

RELAXING OIL BLENDS

Begin by choosing 100 percent therapeutic grade essential oils. Select an organic, unrefined, cold-pressed carrier oil with a complementary scent: sesame, jojoba, sweet almond, coconut, rose hip seed, or olive. Combine oils in a squeeze or pump bottle and roll between palms to blend. Do a skin patch test before applying. Use the following recipes for deep self-love:

WORTHY BLEND:

★ 14 drops bergamot
★ 12 drops sandalwood
★ 6 drops rose

★ 4 drops jasmine
★ 4 drops ylang ylang
★ 4 ounces jojoba

OPEN HEART BLEND:

★ 14 drops lavender
★ 12 drops sweet marjoram

★ 8 drops peppermint
★ 8 drops sweet orange
★ 4 ounces olive oil

9. SACRED OIL ANOINTMENT

Bringing in elements of ancient healing traditions, this ritual involves accessing peaceful rhythms through your pulse points. You will be blessing your body with anointing oils while meditating on your pulse, which is believed to balance the hemispheres of the brain and recalibrate the nervous system for an incredibly calming effect. This practice naturally elicits certain elements of a sleep-friendly experience including mindful attention, self-compassion, and slower breathing.

Follow these steps with care and use the suggested anointing blends to concentrate a scattered mind and promote restorative sleep:

1. Sit in a comfortable position, spine straight. Form your intentions for a peaceful sleep. Speak a blessing over your oil, such as "I ask for your healing energy tonight. Thank you."

2. Dab oil on the first two fingers of each hand and rest them gently on your temples. Close your eyes.

3. Feel for and focus on your pulse for several deep belly breaths. Notice how slower breaths slow the pulse. If you cannot feel your pulse, listen intuitively.

4. Mentally recite a simple mantra in time with your pulse to reaffirm your intention, such as "Peace is in my pulse."

5. Follow this protocol as you move to each pulse point—and a few others, for relaxation's sake—applying gentle pressure: behind the ears, bottom of the throat, on the thumb side of both wrists, inside the elbows, behind the knees, behind the ankles, top of the feet, bottom of the feet.

ANOINTING BLENDS

Crystal-and-oil elixirs offer unique vibrational support for the journey inward. Choose organic essential oils diluted in an unrefined carrier oil: jojoba, olive, sweet almond, rose, and coconut work well. Perform a skin patch test to avoid allergic reactions; keep away from eyes and orifices. As some crystals are toxic infused in liquid, choose some of the following or research others before including.

Method: Combine essential oils and gemstone chips in a 10 ml glass roller bottle or vial. Top with carrier oil. Roll between palms to blend. Anoint pulse points with love.

SACRED EARTH ELIXIR: a grounding blend for whole-body harmony:

- ★ 2 drops Palo Santo
- ★ 2 drops black spruce
- ★ 2 drops cedarwood
- ★ 2 drops cypress
- ★ 2 drops frankincense
- ★ Smoky quartz chips

SACRED SKY ELIXIR: an uplifting blend for spiritual enlightenment:

- ★ 4 drops jasmine
- ★ 3 drops sandalwood
- ★ 2 drops patchouli
- ★ 1 drop German chamomile
- ★ Clear quartz chips

SACRED HEART ELIXIR: a comforting blend for emotional balancing:

- ★ 4 drops lavender
- ★ 2 drops Chinese rose
- ★ 2 drops benzoin (resin oil)
- ★ 2 drops myrrh
- ★ Rose quartz chips

10. OIL PULLING

The mouth is considered to be the mirror into the general health of the body. This is why oil pulling, an age-old remedy rooted in Ayurvedic medicine, is believed to support overall well-being. The process is simple: swish a certain oil in the mouth for 20 minutes. Enjoy fresh breath, whiter teeth, reduced plaque, and potentially a whole host of other benefits as the oil "pulls" bacteria and food particles hiding in crevices and between teeth. Imagine every last bit of your day being extracted, too, clearing away distractions—freshening your mind, strengthening your present-moment awareness, and making space to recharge during tonight's slumber.

Oil pulling in the evening allows for a "moment of silence" as you're winding down from the day; nose breathing naturally cues your body's relaxation response and inspires slower rhythms. By supporting the body's capacity to self-heal, it is a unique and effective way to tune in and take care of yourself.

Go to bed with a fresh, clean feeling in your mouth, and sweet dreams might just be a little bit easier to come by.

Follow the following guidelines for peace and quiet from the inside out:

1. Use 1 teaspoon to 1 tablespoon organic cold-pressed oil— whatever feels best. Sesame oil is the traditional choice, while coconut oil has a milder taste. Avoid using chemically created oils such as soybean, corn, canola, or vegetable oil.

2. Gently swish around your mouth for 20 minutes at the most, starting with 5–10 minutes if you experience any discomfort. The oil will thicken as it mixes with your saliva. Avoid swallowing, as it will also be mixed with bacteria.

3. When finished, spit into a trash can or a paper towel. Don't spit into the sink as the oil can solidify and clog pipes.

4. Thoroughly rinse your mouth with warm water and follow up with tooth brushing.

COCONUT OIL PULLING CHEWS

Try these premade Coconut Oil Pulling Chews using essential oils to make this ritual even more enjoyable (yields 1–2 dozen servings):

★ Melt ½ cup coconut oil on the stovetop or in the microwave in intervals, stirring until liquid. Immediately remove from heat once melted.

★ Add 16–24 drops certified food grade essential oils: cinnamon, clove bud, tea tree, lemon, orange, or peppermint work well.

★ Pour into mini silicone ice cube trays or candy molds and put in the fridge for about 45 minutes or the freezer for about 30 minutes to harden.

★ Remove from trays and store in an airtight container in the fridge. Virgin, unrefined coconut oil will last months, even years; refer to the "best by" date.

★ Use 1–2 chews nightly for pulling (depending on molds used and preferred serving size), following the same guidelines for regular pulling.

11. BOAR BRISTLE BRUSHING

Care for your hair the old-fashioned way with a boar bristle brush and you'll see why this ritual has lasted centuries. Being almost identical to human hair in texture, boar bristles effectively redistribute your scalp's natural oils, alleviating oily roots and conditioning dry ends. A soft, protective, healthful shine isn't the only benefit you'll notice: the stimulating scalp massage and gentle stretch feels utterly divine at the end of a long day. Enjoying a few relaxing minutes of brushing before bed is an act of self-care, a moment carved out of the night for nurturing.

Brushing is best done with a 100 percent natural boar bristle brush, which you can find online or in health stores. The style of brush and the time this ritual takes depends on the texture of your hair. A pure boar bristle brush is best for thin, straight hair while a brush with a mixture of nylon and boar bristles works well for thick, curly hair.

Brush nightly for best results—not just for the health of your hair but as a means of transitioning into a meditative state. While you're performing this ritual, meditate on how your hair is appreciating being clothed in nature's best conditioning elixir: its own oils, and your loving attention. Enjoy the sedating massage. Savor the stretch. Embrace the moment.

With your hair completely dry, begin this unwinding ceremony:

1. Gently work out any tangles with your fingers or a wide-tooth comb, using oils of almond, avocado, or jojoba to assist.

2. With brush in hand, carefully fold forward from the hips with a long torso, knees slightly bent for comfort. Enjoy this

gentle stretch. Consider the postural elements of Standing Forward Fold (see Chapter 5).

3. Brush from the nape of your neck, working in gentle strokes from root to tip for 3–5 minutes. After a few brush strokes, your hair will become supple and cooperative. If you encounter tangles while brushing, stop to detangle.

4. Root through your feet, engage your core, draw your tailbone down, and inhale with a flat back as you slowly return to standing.

5. Run your brush, now filled with sebaceous oil, from the crown of your head down to the ends for 3–5 minutes. If you have thick or curly hair, part into sections with soft cloth bands or clips.

6. Repeat this process twice.

7. If desired, rub a few drops of oil into ends and leave in overnight for additional nourishment.

Clean your brush regularly, using a comb to carefully remove hair and product build-up. Rinse bristles under warm water and gently cleanse with a natural shampoo. Squeeze any excess water from the cushion. Lay with bristles facing down on a towel to dry overnight.

12. BOTANICAL DREAM EYE PILLOW

When you desperately need some respite—and personal space—take a mini-vacation and slip away underneath the gentle weight of a dream pillow. Laying a pillow over your eyes induces a feeling of safety and calm, blocks sleep-disrupting light, and can ease tension headaches. They are perfect for bed, reclining yoga poses, and some meditations and visualizations.

This basic eye pillow tutorial uses naturally cool flaxseed infused with an aromatherapeutic blend of lavender, chamomile, rose, and hops to promote deep sleep. Prepare to escape the rest of the world and sink into a long moment of serenity. Tired eyes will thank you and let the rest of your body know that it's time to de-stress.

You will need:

★ ¾ cup flaxseed

★ ¼ cup herbs: 2 parts each dried lavender flowers and rose petals, 1 part each dried chamomile flowers and hops (or your own blend)

★ Measuring cup

★ 4–5 drops lavender essential oil (optional)

★ Fabric cut to a 9" square: silk, satin, cotton, flannel

★ Iron (optional)

★ Thread, needle, and scissors

Instructions:

1. Mix flaxseed and herbs in a measuring cup. Add essential oil drops if desired.

2. If not already, cut your selected fabric into a 9" square. Iron fabric if needed.

3. If your fabric frays easily, sew a ¼" zig-zag pattern around the entire edge.

4. Fold the fabric in half with the "wrong side" (inside of the pillow) facing out. Now you will have a rectangular shape that is beginning to look like an eye pillow.

5. Sew a tight ½" seam around the fabric, leaving a 2" opening on one side.

6. Fold the pillow right side out through the opening. Press seams with iron (optional).

7. Fill pillow with your herbal blend.

8. Fold the opening in and sew closed.

9. Gently massage the pillow to distribute contents. Scent will last for several months, even years.

For more protection, make an additional washable pillow casing (using a 10" square) to cover the pillow you just made. Follow steps 2 through 6 and leave one shorter side completely open for easy removal of inner pillow. To wash, treat as a delicate fabric.

Explore your favorite materials and blends scented with sleep in mind: wormwood, cloves, catnip, lemon balm, mugwort, calendula flowers, and gemstone chips also make lovely dream pillows.

DREAMY SLEEP SACHETS

While you're feeling crafty, fill a cotton muslin bag or make your own herbal sachets from scratch:

★ Cut two identically-shaped pieces of fabric.

★ Align fabric pieces on top of each other and sew together.

★ Before finishing the stitch, fill with desired blend: 1–2 tablespoons dried herbs, crystal chips, 5–8 drops essential oils. Sew closed.

★ Place inside, under, or next to pillows.

13. FACE YOGA

Face yoga coordinates simple facial exercises, massage, acupressure, and relaxation to soften the accumulation of stress in your face, neck, and shoulders. A few minutes of this sleep sequence can ease tension headaches, calm the mind, boost self-esteem, bring inner and outer radiance, lessen chronic pain, and improve your quality of sleep. Some elements of Sukshma yoga are included to soothe facial muscles and nerve connections. You will look *and feel* more relaxed.

Instructions:

1. Sit or stand in front of a mirror. Be kind with what you see.
2. Place your index finger between your eyebrows with gentle pressure. Close your eyes. Take a few deep nose breaths. Circle your finger in one direction, then the other.
3. Place both index fingers at the beginning (inner edge) of your eyebrows. Make gentle circles across the tops of your eyebrows. Follow the bone around your eyes, ending at the bridge of your nose.
4. Bring both index fingers to the inner orbit of each eye at the edge of the nose with gentle pressure. Eyes closed, breathe deeply. Circle your fingers in both directions.
5. Rub your palms together to generate heat. Cup them over your closed eyes. Take a few deep breaths.
6. Place both index fingers on your temples with gentle pressure. Eyes closed, breathe deeply. Circle your fingers in both directions.

7. Place your index fingers on either side of the nostrils with gentle pressure. Breathe. Circle your fingers in both directions.

8. Rest all fingers at the center of your forehead and stroke them horizontally with a feather-light touch, sweeping (not dragging) off the sides. Repeat ten times.

9. Gently pinch all around the cheeks and jawline.

10. Use your thumbs to gently sweep up the jawline a few times.

11. With your thumbs and index fingers, gently and slowly pull the earlobes downward a few times for a total of 30 seconds. Pull them outward, then rotate them in both directions—30 seconds each.

12. Place your hands and all fingers on the neck. Tilt the chin slightly and stroke down to your collarbone a few times. With hands resting on your collarbone, stick your bottom lip out as much as you can, feeling the neck muscle working.

13. Place your index finger at the center of your collarbone with gentle pressure. Breathe. Circle your finger in both directions.

14. Simply close your eyes and smile very slightly (like the Buddha). Relax the rest of the face completely. Breathe deeply for a few moments or minutes.

15. Place your index finger at the top of your head with gentle pressure. Close your eyes. Take a few (or more) deep breaths before releasing the practice.

——— CHAPTER 4 ———

CONSCIOUS CONSUMPTION

A thriving ecosystem contributes to restful sleep and relief from ailments. Each of the recipes in this chapter features simple, nutritious ingredients to support the body's natural nighttime repair process. They are light and accessible, not excessive (since too much of anything before bed can interrupt your dreamy vibes). To ensure you receive all your *Zzzz's*, sip the last of your caffeine around noon and eat dinner 3–4 hours before bedtime, keeping spicy foods, nicotine, and alcohol to a minimum (or nonexistent). See how it feels to dedicate the last hours of your day to nourishment. You might be surprised by how transformative this time can be.

You might also be pleasantly surprised by how you feel when you love how you eat—not guilty, bloated, or deprived but alive and connected. Craft a wholly enriching experience with each nighttime snack, using the following notes as a guide.

For your kitchen:

★ Use decor that makes you smile. String fairy lights. Play soft music. Light candles. Minimize distractions (phone, television).

★ Choose soothing colors for tableware such as blue or lavender. Reserve special tableware for evening rituals. Sit down at a table.

★ Only engage in heart-nurturing conversation—nothing stressful.

★ Appreciate the time you spend here preparing something meaningful. Savor the slow process as much as the end product.

For your body:

★ Consult the feelings underneath your cravings. Ask yourself, "Would this feel nurturing?" Take conscious care of yourself.

★ Practice full belly breaths.

★ Let positive emotions flood your body. Place your hands on your heart and belly. Affirm your worth. Thank your body.

★ Soften: shoulders, eyes, forehead. Feel your feet on the floor.

For your food:

★ Look at your food. Notice every color, texture, smell, flavor.
★ Thank your food. Honor its life energy. Celebrate nature's abundance.
★ Chew until dissolved before swallowing—even liquids. Give your brain time to catch up with your belly. Give your belly a break. Receive the nutrients.
★ Document every sensation and delight in a food journal (optional).

To eat and sleep peacefully, live in the moment. Let your awareness and the evening grow expansive. You will go to bed feeling fulfilled.

1. CHERRY SWIRLED BANANA NUT TOAST

One of the best ways to sleep like a dream is to go back to the basics. Though an ordinary slice of toast may not seem like an ingredient for a ritual, read on and watch it be transformed into a near-magical creation. Tart cherry–swirled yogurt spread on whole grain toast and topped with banana slices, crushed pistachios, pumpkin seeds, and a drizzle of almond butter gives you everything you need to chew your way into a sleepy state of mind.

No need for pre-flavored yogurt—you'll be swirling in tart cherry concentrate for a hearty dose of the sleep-time hormone melatonin. Anti-inflammatory properties dance with the potassium and magnesium in the banana slices to relax your muscles and nerves. A drizzle of almond butter, crushed pistachios, and a sprinkle of pumpkin seeds add just the right amount of protein, B vitamins, and magnesium to promote your rest-and-digest cycle and maintain a stable blood sugar level while sleeping. Finally, bring it all together on a slice of whole grain toast, which cues the temporary release of insulin followed by the key calming hormones tryptophan and serotonin.

Upgrading your toast in a loving fashion communicates to your body that it is time to prepare for sleep. While you can use tart cherry juice for this recipe, the concentrate offers not just a thicker consistency but also a higher concentration of melatonin. Enjoy turning the familiar into a tasty new way to call in sweet slumber.

This recipe yields 2 servings.

Ingredients:

- ★ 2 slices whole grain bread
- ★ 4 tablespoons plain unsweetened yogurt (Greek, skyr, or plant-based)
- ★ 1 tablespoon Montmorency tart cherry concentrate
- ★ 1 medium banana, sliced
- ★ 1 tablespoon crushed pistachios (about 8 whole pistachios, shells removed)
- ★ 1 tablespoon pumpkin seeds
- ★ 1 tablespoon melted almond butter

Instructions:

1. Set bread to toast. While your bread is toasting, add yogurt to a small bowl and fold in tart cherry concentrate for a swirled appearance.
2. Spread tart cherry yogurt onto each piece of toast.
3. Top with banana slices.
4. Sprinkle on crushed pistachios and pumpkin seeds, and drizzle on almond butter.
5. Serve immediately on a pastel-colored plate for soothing vibes.

Allow each creamy and crunchy bite to lull you into a more relaxed state. Imagine all the elements of this humble snack working together to induce sleep from the inside out.

2. MAPLE CRUNCH YOGURT

Magnesium-rich nuts and seeds are caramelized in pure maple syrup and molasses, then married with warming spices and a touch of sea salt for a satisfying crunch that sets the stage for easy sleep. The natural sugars provide a slight insulin boost to prevent sleep-disrupting sugar spikes. Tart cherries offer a dose of melatonin and apricot helps your body recover from stress. All of this combined with the healthy fats, vitamins, and minerals in yogurt, and you're in for a real treat. Your nerves, muscles, heart, and belly will thank you for this anything-but-ordinary bowl of bedtime bliss.

Enjoy this perfect marriage of salty and sweet about 1–2 hours before bedtime. You might just be one crunchy dessert away from better sleep.

This recipe yields 6 "maple crunch" servings.

Ingredients:

- ★ ½ teaspoon ground cinnamon
- ★ ¼ teaspoon ground nutmeg
- ★ ¼ teaspoon ground cardamom
- ★ ⅛ teaspoon vanilla extract
- ★ ⅛ teaspoon sea salt
- ★ ⅔ cup walnuts
- ★ ⅓ cup sliced almonds
- ★ ⅓ cup pumpkin seeds
- ★ 3 tablespoons sunflower seeds
- ★ ⅓ cup pure maple syrup
- ★ 2 teaspoons molasses
- ★ ⅓ cup dried Montmorency cherries
- ★ ⅓ cup dried apricots
- ★ 1 cup organic plain unsweetened yogurt (Greek, skyr, or plant-based)

Instructions:

1. Line a rimmed baking sheet with parchment paper. Set aside.

2. Mix cinnamon, nutmeg, cardamom, vanilla, salt, walnuts, almonds, pumpkin seeds, and sunflower seeds in a medium bowl. Set aside.

3. Add maple syrup and molasses to a large saucepan and heat over medium heat until just beginning to simmer.

4. Add your mixture of spices, nuts, and seeds. Stir frequently, until syrup has reduced (about 3–5 minutes).

5. Spread mixture evenly on the prepared baking sheet. Sprinkle on dried fruit and stir until evenly distributed, breaking up clusters as needed. Let cool completely.

6. Add ½ cup mixture to 1 cup yogurt. Enjoy in your favorite mug or heart-shaped bowl.

7. Store remaining "maple crunch" mixture in an airtight container for up to a week.

MAPLE CRUNCH FROZEN YOGURT BITES

For a frozen treat that hits the sweet-and-salty spot on warm nights (yields 4–8 servings):

★ Mix 2 cups yogurt and 2 cups "maple crunch" into an 8" × 8" glass baking dish lined with tinfoil. Spread evenly.

★ Freeze until firm.

★ Remove frozen yogurt spread from dish by gently pulling out tinfoil.

★ Carefully slice into 8 squares and store in an airtight container in the freezer.

★ Enjoy 1–2 squares for dessert.

---

3. COMFORTING RICE PUDDING

Made with sleep in mind and enjoyed about 4 hours before bedtime, this creamy, Comforting Rice Pudding is a golden ticket to Dreamland. Jasmine rice shortens the amount of time it takes to transition from wakefulness to sleep, possibly due to the boosted levels of tryptophan and serotonin, two brain chemicals involved in sleep. Cook it up fluffy right in milk alongside warming spices and a few of nature's favorite sweeteners, and you have all the indulgence of a comfort food without the guilt. Top with melatonin-rich cherry concentrate and sleep-promoting nuts for a beloved treat.

While this recipe features aromatic rice for a unique flavor and a perfectly creamy texture, you can certainly experiment with other varieties, such as brown rice for a thicker, chewy consistency and its own nutritional profile (which includes sleep-promoting melatonin and B vitamins).

This recipe yields 4–6 servings.

Ingredients:

★ 1 cup full-fat coconut milk from can
★ 1 cup brown or white jasmine rice (alternatives: basmati, Arborio, brown)
★ 1 cinnamon stick
★ ⅛ teaspoon sea salt
★ 1 cup milk of choice (cow, coconut, almond), divided
★ ¼ cup maple syrup
★ ½ teaspoon ground nutmeg
★ ½ teaspoon vanilla extract
★ ¼ teaspoon almond extract

- ★ 6 Medjool dates, seeded and chopped into raisin-sized pieces
- ★ For topping: drizzle Montmorency tart cherry concentrate, dash ground cinnamon, sprinkling slivered almonds or chopped walnuts (optional)

Instructions:

1. In a medium nonstick saucepan with a heavy bottom, bring 1 cup full-fat coconut milk to a gentle boil. While warming, rinse and drain the rice well.

2. Reduce heat to simmer. Add rice, cinnamon stick, salt, and ½ cup milk of choice (cow, coconut, almond).

3. Simmer for 10–15 minutes covered, stirring frequently to make sure the rice does not stick. Mixture will gradually thicken.

4. In a small mixing bowl, combine remaining ½ cup milk, maple syrup, nutmeg, vanilla and almond extracts, and chopped dates.

5. When most of the liquid has absorbed in the saucepan, add contents of your mixing bowl.

6. Cover and simmer for another 10–15 minutes, stirring frequently until most of the liquid is absorbed.

7. Test a spoonful to see if the texture and taste is to your liking. If needed, add a splash more milk and a sprinkle of any seasonings to taste. Simmer uncovered until ready.

8. Remove from heat. Remove cinnamon stick.

9. Spoon into your favorite bowls or mugs and let cool before enjoying. Sprinkle or drizzle any desired toppings.

10. Store leftovers in airtight containers in the fridge up to 4 days. Reheat on the stove with a splash of milk.

4. OVEN-ROASTED CHICKPEAS

Keep a can of these tasty nut alternatives, also known as garbanzo beans, in your kitchen cupboard to satisfy crunchy cravings after dinner. These little legumes are a rich source of vitamin B_6, an essential vitamin for the production of the sleep hormone melatonin, and provide the body with a much-needed dose of magnesium to support relaxation and restful nights. A little time in the oven and you might just meet your new favorite snack. The crunchy texture is even more satisfying when you enjoy the process of exploring your favorite flavors.

Due to their high protein content, roasted chickpeas are best enjoyed a few hours before bedtime. There are endless possibilities; begin with one of the following recipes to ensure you're making a sleep-friendly treat.

This recipe yields 2–3 servings.

Ingredients:

★ 1 (15-ounce) can chickpeas, or 2 cups

SALT AND PEPPER CHICKPEAS:

★ 2¼ teaspoons olive oil

★ ¼ teaspoon sea salt, or to taste

★ ¼ teaspoon ground black pepper, or to taste

HONEY CINNAMON CHICKPEAS:

★ ½ tablespoon coconut oil

★ ¼ teaspoon ground cinnamon

★ ⅛ teaspoon ground nutmeg

★ 2 tablespoons raw honey

★ ⅛ teaspoon sea salt (optional)

PARMESAN ROSEMARY CHICKPEAS:

- ★ 1 tablespoon olive oil
- ★ 1 tablespoon nutritional yeast
- ★ 1 teaspoon crushed rosemary
- ★ ¼ teaspoon sea salt, or to taste

SESAME SEED CHICKPEAS:

- ★ 2¼ teaspoons sesame oil
- ★ 1 tablespoon sesame seeds
- ★ ¼ teaspoon sea salt, or to taste

Instructions:

1. Preheat the oven to 400°F.
2. Line a baking sheet with parchment paper. Set aside.
3. Drain and rinse chickpeas.
4. Spread on a paper towel to dry. Pat dry with a paper towel to remove as much moisture as possible.
5. Spread dried chickpeas in a single layer on the baking sheet.
6. Bake for 25–40 minutes, shaking the pan or stirring every 10 minutes until crispy. When you have a crispy and golden exterior with a buttery interior, remove from oven.
7. Transfer warm chickpeas to a medium mixing bowl and drizzle with oil. Sprinkle on desired seasonings and toss until coated. Add extra oil, if necessary.
8. Return to oven for another 5 minutes to let mixture absorb (and for the honey cinnamon flavor to caramelize), checking often to ensure you have your desired texture without burning.
9. Remove and let cool before enjoying. Store leftovers in an airtight container at room temperature up to 1 week. Warm in the oven at 300°F for a few minutes to re-crisp.

5. SPICED VEGAN "BUTTER" POPCORN

Homemade stovetop popcorn is an easy, quick, and inexpensive way to turn an ordinary night into a moment worth savoring. The complex carbohydrates stimulate the slow release of sleepy serotonin without loading your system with calories, making it an ideal bedtime snack when made healthfully. Enjoy the process of creating a fluffy bowl of vegan goodness—you won't miss the butter (or the chemicals) and you can keep your happy crunch while benefiting from the enhanced nutritional profile.

You may not find nutritional yeast in your kitchen cabinet on a regular basis. Find this "cheesy" alternative online or in most health food sections: flaky and powdery versions are rich with B-complex vitamins, dairy-free, gluten-free, and vegan (be sure to read brand labels).

Anti-inflammatory turmeric, sweet cinnamon, a dash of salt and pepper, and coconut oil form a light, "buttery" treat that's best savored at least 1 hour before bedtime.

This recipe yields 3–4 servings (about 8 cups).

Before you begin, have the following kitchenware ready to go:

★ 1 large saucepan with lid
★ 1 small mixing bowl
★ 1 small glass bowl or microwave-safe container
★ 1 large mixing bowl or rimmed baking sheet
★ 1 mixing spoon

Ingredients:

★ ¼ cup nutritional yeast
★ 1 teaspoon Himalayan salt
★ 1 teaspoon ground cinnamon
★ 1 teaspoon turmeric powder
★ ⅛ teaspoon black pepper

- ★ 2 tablespoons coconut oil (optional, for drizzling)
- ★ 2 tablespoons coconut oil (to coat the bottom of the pan)
- ★ ½ cup fresh organic popcorn kernels (fresh pops best)

Instructions:

1. Combine nutritional yeast, salt, and spices in a small mixing bowl. Set aside.

2. If using, heat 2 tablespoons coconut oil in a microwave-safe container, removing every 10 seconds to stir until melted. Set aside.

3. Melt the other 2 tablespoons coconut oil in a large, covered saucepan on medium heat. Once oil has completely melted, add two individual kernels to the oil and cover.

4. When kernels pop, uncover and add the rest of the popcorn to form a single layer on the bottom of the pan. Cover and shake to coat kernels with oil.

5. Carefully monitor the popcorn. When popping begins, shake the pan every 10 seconds or so to prevent burning.

6. When popping slows to a pop every few seconds, remove the pan from heat and continue to shake until popping subsides.

7. Immediately pour popcorn into a large mixing bowl or rimmed baking sheet. Drizzle with optional melted coconut oil, and sprinkle your seasonings. Shake well or toss to coat with a mixing spoon, adding more seasonings to taste.

6. OVEN-BAKED VEGGIE CHIPS

When you have "crunchy" on your mind, skip the bag of chips and reach for a sweet potato or a bunch of kale instead (or both). Sweet potatoes are a great source of complex carbohydrates, potassium, magnesium, and calcium to help you relax and sleep better. Sliced and lightly kissed with seasoned oil and then baked to crispy perfection, they're a treat all on their own.

Praised for its superfood qualities, kale delivers a healthy dose of sleep-supporting potassium, calcium, vitamin B_6, and magnesium. Apple cider vinegar and nutritional yeast offer a unique flavor without the guilt of store-bought chips.

Enjoyed on separate occasions or brought together, these two versatile veggies create a delightful experience worth sharing—but beware the temptation not to share. Sharing is caring.

This recipe yields 2–4 servings.

Ingredients for sweet potato chips:

★ 2 medium organically grown sweet potatoes

★ 2 tablespoons olive or coconut oil

★ ¼ teaspoon each salt and pepper, or to taste

★ Optional seasonings: 1 teaspoon thyme or rosemary

Instructions for sweet potato chips:

1. Preheat oven to 350°F.

2. Wash sweet potatoes and peel off the skin, if desired (not necessary if organic, but remove if conventionally grown).

3. Slice sweet potatoes into even, thin rounds—thicker for sturdier chips, thinner for crispy chips. Use a mandoline slicer for ease and speed, or use a knife to slice by hand.

4. In a medium bowl, toss with oil, salt and pepper, and seasonings until lightly coated on all sides.

5. Arrange in a single layer on baking sheets lined with parchment paper.

6. Bake until golden and edges start to curl on one side (about 10–15 minutes) then flip to ensure evenness—thicker slices will take longer.

7. Remove and let cool before eating.

Ingredients for kale chips:

★ 1 large bunch kale (not baby kale)

★ 1 tablespoon apple cider vinegar

★ ½ tablespoon avocado oil

★ 2 tablespoons nutritional yeast

★ ½ teaspoon sea salt, or to taste

Instructions for kale chips:

1. Preheat oven to 350°F.

2. Tear kale off stalks and into large bite-size pieces (will shrink slightly while baking).

3. Wash and dry, using a salad spinner or patting with a paper towel.

4. In a large bowl, drizzle vinegar and oil and massage into leaves until soft and slightly darker. Sprinkle nutritional yeast and salt and massage to distribute.

5. Arrange in a single layer on baking sheets lined with parchment paper.

6. Bake about 8–12 minutes until crispy.

7. Remove and let cool before eating.

7. SWEET DREAMY "NICE" CREAM

Not merely a healthy substitute for artificially-sweetened ice cream, this after-dinner dessert is a delightful treat in its own right—and it is fantastically easy to create. The essentials: frozen bananas. Rich with sleep-inducing potassium and magnesium, bananas are natural muscle relaxants and can help prevent painful cramping in the middle of the night. Plus, watching the blender magically morph them into a dreamy, creamy confection might cause you to change the way you look at your food. Feel a shift in perspective coming on as you turn regular old bananas into a nighttime ritual you can't help but look forward to.

This naturally sweet one-ingredient treat can be elevated with a dash of warming spices, melatonin-rich cherries or almond butter, or a sprinkle of soothing lavender or rose powder to help lull your body into a harmonious slumber. Start simple and have fun exploring mix-ins and add-ons as you whip up something special for yourself tonight.

This recipe yields 4 servings. (Cut recipe in half for small blenders.)

Ingredients:

- ★ 4 large ripe bananas
- ★ 1–2 tablespoons plant-based milk (optional)
- ★ Mix-ins: 2 tablespoons almond butter; handful Montmorency cherries with ¼ teaspoon rose powder; handful blueberries with ¼ teaspoon lavender powder; ⅛ teaspoon each cardamom and cinnamon (all optional)
- ★ Toppings: raw honey; melted almond butter; Montmorency tart cherry concentrate (optional)

Instructions:

1. Peel bananas and slice into thin discs.
2. Arrange on a baking sheet or large plate and freeze 1–2 hours (or until you're ready to use).
3. Remove banana slices from freezer and let thaw about 15 minutes.
4. Puree in a powerful blender or food processor until smooth and creamy. Take breaks to scrape down the sides when they stick. If needed, add 1–2 tablespoons plant-based milk to ease the process.
5. When you have a nice, creamy consistency that resembles ice cream, add desired mix-ins and blend just until mixed through and smooth.
6. Serve immediately with desired toppings.

If you happen to over-blend, simply refreeze and blend again. Freeze any leftovers and re-blend when you are ready to serve—always allow frozen ingredients to thaw a bit before blending, breaking up with a spoon as needed.

Prepare for sleep knowing that you were kind to your body tonight. You chose to look at your food as nourishment, not punishment. Ponder how amazing nature is for offering a single ingredient that can be reshaped into a beloved moment of bliss. This is what loving your body looks and feels like.

8. ROSE PETAL INFUSED HONEY

If you just can't sleep without a little nighttime sweet, you might as well delight in an easy treat that not only tastes divine but results in sweet dreams. While a spoonful of honey can do the trick, Rose Petal Infused Honey makes you feel luxurious (and calm) without requiring much effort on your part. As its delicate aroma lifts your spirits and comforts the heart, rest assured that you are making something special that your body will thank you for later.

The humble rose has long been adored for its ability to reduce nervous tension, ease sadness, calm heart palpitations, eliminate liver congestion, and reduce inflammation. Tranquility and love will be two qualities you notice sinking into your being, turning an otherwise ordinary evening into a heavenly retreat.

Receive the aesthetic, physiological, and spiritual gifts of enjoying Rose Petal Infused Honey as a nightly ritual. There are so many ways to bask in the beauty of this special creation. Enjoy a spoonful or add to your evening tea, warm milk, oatmeal, plain yogurt, whole grain toast, "nice" cream, bath, or face mask when you need a little lift.

This recipe will yield any serving size of your choice.

You will need:

★ Glass jar with lid (any size will do, depending on how much you want to make)

★ Enough fresh or dried organic, edible rose petals to fill your jar (only use petals you are sure haven't been sprayed with chemicals)

* ★ Raw local honey to fill jar
* ★ Stirring stick
* ★ Bowl of warm water to liquefy honey, if needed

Instructions:

1. Gather enough rose petals (fresh or dried) to fill your jar. If using fresh, harvest after dew has evaporated and before heated by midday sun. Petals should be dry and free of dust.

2. Fill your jar with rose petals. The jar should not be too spacious or packed too tightly.

3. Pour liquefied honey over the rose petals until completely covered. You may need to place your jar of honey in a bowl of warm water to liquefy first—do not let honey boil if using another method of heating as it will destroy the enzymes.

4. Stir rose petals and honey to release any air bubbles until well-combined. Pour more honey in as needed to fill the jar.

5. Cover with a tight-fitting lid. Allow to infuse in a cool, dry place for a few days before using, turning upside down a couple times each day. This mixture will last indefinitely, but feel free to store in the fridge in warm weather.

6. Serve the honey with the petals for full benefits and an exquisite experience.

9. SERENDIPITEA

Drinking herbal tea before bedtime is an age-old practice for soothing yourself to sleep—and one you are likely familiar with. Certain herbs ease anxiety and depression, promote relaxation, release muscle tension, and improve quality of sleep. Not only that, but the ceremonial act of preparing a cup of tea can be a highly spiritual experience. As you slow down to savor the present moment and the simple practice of making a beloved beverage, you become an energetic match for sleep. With simplicity comes tranquility: sweet serendipity.

Enjoy this tea ritual 1–2 hours before bedtime.

This recipe yields 1 serving.

Ingredients:

★ 1 cup water or organic milk
★ 1 heaping teaspoon decaffeinated tea (see following suggestions)
★ 1 tablespoon collagen peptides, grass-fed ghee, coconut oil, or MCT oil (optional)
★ 1 teaspoon raw honey (optional)
★ ⅛ teaspoon vanilla extract (optional)

Instructions:

1. Craft a cozy environment with dim lighting, soft music, blankets, and so on. Let this be a moment of indulgence.
2. Bring water or milk to a boil in your kettle or saucepan.
3. Intuitively choose your tea blend. Enjoy the anticipation of drinking your tea. Listen to the bubbling of the liquid. Take deep breaths.

4. When water or milk is boiling, turn off heat. Add 1 heaping teaspoon of your tea blend (in a mesh strainer, if you have one) to the milk, or pour water over your tea into a teapot or mug. If you are making a pot of tea, add an extra teaspoon "for the pot." Steep 5–20 minutes.

5. Observe the slowly changing color as if the liquid is being infused with the energy of sleep.

6. When steeped, strain any loose leaves and pour into a favorite mug with care.

7. Mix in desired optional ingredients until dissolved. Imagine you are mixing in the very essence of peace.

8. Wrap your hands around the mug. Absorb its warmth, scent, taste, and calming properties. Bask in this moment you have set aside for yourself.

HERBAL TEA BLENDS

Herbs perfect for a sleepy-time blend: calendula flowers, chamomile flowers, hibiscus flowers, hops flowers, lavender flowers, lemon balm leaf, mugwort leaf, passionflower, peppermint leaf, rose petals, skullcap leaf, St. John's wort, valerian root.

Experiment with these other favorite blends:

★ Soothes belly and mind: 4 parts each lemon balm leaf, peppermint leaf, chamomile flowers, plus 1 part passionflower

★ Comforts the heart: 8 parts rose petals, 2 parts chamomile flowers, 1 part each lavender flowers, calendula flowers, skullcap leaf

★ Ultimate sedative: 8 parts each chamomile flowers, lemon balm leaf, skullcap leaf, plus 4 parts mugwort leaf, plus 2 parts lavender flowers, plus 1 part each hops flowers, valerian root

Method: Mix herbs in a large bowl. Store mixture in an airtight glass container in a cool, dry place. Use within 6 months.

10. LAVENDER CHERRY MOON MILK

A heavenly treat, this Lavender Cherry Moon Milk is made to be a cherished bedtime ritual. The creamy and calming beverage highlights tart cherries, lavender flowers, and plant-based milk for a truly lovely blend. The result is nothing short of comfort—a subtly sweet cup of nourishment that's perfect for when you need a little extra support.

Tart cherries are one of the few natural sources of melatonin, the sleep hormone that regulates your body's internal clock. Also containing sleep-inducing tryptophan and serotonin, cherries are a powerful fruit that will help you sleep more soundly and wake fewer times throughout the night. Nibble on a few fresh cherries when in season and incorporate them (or their juice) into a warm lunar beverage for something quite spectacular.

Lavender makes a welcome appearance in this recipe for its calming, healing properties and its ability to promote sleep. You can grow lavender in your garden or find dried, edible flowers at your local or online health food store. As you become more and more familiar with recreating this ritual, you can experiment with other herbs, such as rose petals.

With its roots in Ayurvedic medicine, this moon milk recipe is made to be vegan, though you can use organic grass-fed cow's milk or substitute raw honey for maple syrup. Enjoy this enchanting creation about 1–2 hours before bedtime and settle in for a good, peaceful rest.

This recipe yields 1 serving.

Ingredients:

- ★ 1 cup plant-based milk of choice
- ★ ⅓ cup pitted Montmorency tart cherries, fresh or frozen, or ⅓ cup 100% tart cherry juice
- ★ 2 tablespoons coconut milk from can, or coconut manna
- ★ ½ teaspoon dried edible lavender flowers
- ★ ⅛ teaspoon vanilla extract
- ★ Pinch Himalayan sea salt
- ★ 2 teaspoons pure maple syrup
- ★ 1 tablespoon unrefined coconut oil or MCT oil
- ★ For garnish: crushed dried lavender flowers, dash ground nutmeg (optional)

Instructions:

1. In a food processor or blender combine all ingredients except for coconut or MCT oil.
2. In a small pot, heat blended ingredients over medium heat until near-simmering, whisking until frothy and warmed through.
3. Turn off heat and whisk in coconut or MCT oil.
4. Pour into your favorite mug. For an aromatic finishing touch, lightly sprinkle with crushed dried lavender flowers and ground nutmeg.

In place of dried lavender flowers, you can steep a strong ½ cup of lavender herbal tea using multiple store-bought tea bags. If all of your ingredients are liquid, you can omit blending, but keep if you prefer the drink more foamy. This even makes for a delicious cold beverage on warmer evenings—simply place in the fridge after heating.

11. NUTMEG–SPICED WARM MILK

Offering a trifecta of wholesome goodness, drink this elixir to fall asleep, stay asleep, and wake up feeling refreshed.

The featured ingredient in this delightful mix is ground nutmeg, a well-loved kitchen spice that's commonly used in holiday recipes. Nutmeg is associated with promising health benefits, including its ability to relieve pain, reduce stress, support the immune system, soothe indigestion, detox the body, and induce and increase the duration of sleep. While too much nutmeg can be highly toxic, ¼ teaspoon or less serves as a powerful natural sedative.

Another friend of sleep is unfiltered raw honey. The sweet nectar contains the essential amino acid tryptophan, which activates the release of serotonin, the neurotransmitter that promotes feelings of relaxation, calm, and sleepiness. This "happy hormone" is needed for the production of melatonin, the "hormone of darkness" that regulates sleep and wakefulness. Raw honey may also support liver function. Taken before bed, it fuels the liver, sending a message to the brain that it's being nourished and is safe to rest, thus helping you sleep more soundly and recover faster. A small amount (1–2 teaspoons) of honey before bedtime will do.

Mix together nutmeg and raw honey in a warm mug of milk, and this recipe might be one of the easiest, tastiest nighttime remedies you'll try.

This recipe yields 1 serving.

Ingredients:

★ 1 cup organic grass-fed milk (non-dairy options: almond, rice, coconut)

- ★ ¼ teaspoon ground nutmeg
- ★ 1 teaspoon unfiltered raw honey

Instructions:

1. **Microwave:** Warm up the milk in your favorite mug until a touch hotter than you would comfortably drink. Stir in honey until dissolved. Whisk in ground nutmeg about 30 seconds, until well blended.

2. **Stovetop:** Combine milk and nutmeg in a small saucepan over low heat. Bring to a simmer, whisking frequently, being careful not to let the milk boil. Turn off heat, stir in honey until dissolved, and pour into your favorite mug.

3. Let mixture cool to a comfortable temperature for sipping. Enjoy at least 1 hour before bedtime.

OPTIONAL INGREDIENTS

Experiment with other healthy additions to make this recipe your own: consider any of the following ingredients.

- ★ 1 tablespoon ghee (clarified grass-fed butter)
- ★ 1 tablespoon collagen peptides
- ★ ⅛ teaspoon ground cinnamon
- ★ ⅛ teaspoon turmeric (add a pinch of black pepper for absorption)
- ★ Tiny pinch cardamom
- ★ Splash pure vanilla extract
- ★ 2 tablespoons coconut milk from can

12. NIGHTTIME TURMERIC LATTE

The distinctly golden hue of this spicy beverage is a welcome sight when you experience just how delicious and healthful it is. It's a wonderful way to consume the powerful anti-inflammatory properties of turmeric. With an earthy taste that pairs perfectly with warming ginger and cinnamon, turmeric isn't just great for joint pain—it aids digestion and regulates blood sugar levels to keep you from waking in the middle of the night. Long used to treat depression and insomnia, it makes for a completely heart-warming bedtime tonic.

Take note that turmeric can easily stain kitchenware, countertops, and skin, though not permanently. The color will eventually fade; a little scrubbing with soap or baking soda and water will help.

Adding a little cozy to your evening is easy: sip slowly from your favorite big mug and savor how good it feels to show your body some love. For a heartier drink, you can swap out the milk for grass-fed bone broth.

This recipe yields 1 serving.

Ingredients:

- ★ 1 cup plant-based milk of choice
- ★ ½ teaspoon ground turmeric
- ★ ⅛ teaspoon ground cinnamon
- ★ Pinch ground black pepper
- ★ ⅛ teaspoon ground ginger or fresh peeled ginger
- ★ ⅛ teaspoon ground cloves
- ★ ¼ teaspoon vanilla extract
- ★ 1 teaspoon organic unrefined coconut oil
- ★ 1 teaspoon raw honey or pure maple syrup, or to taste

Instructions:

1. Combine all ingredients except for coconut oil and honey/maple syrup in a blender and pulse until mixed through.

2. In a small saucepan, gently heat blended ingredients over medium-low heat, leisurely whisking for about 5 minutes until near simmering (not boiling).

3. Turn off heat and whisk in coconut oil and honey/maple syrup until frothy.

4. Pour into a large mug and drink immediately.

PREMADE TURMERIC LATTE MIX

For easier nightly preparation and fewer dirty dishes, keep a premade powdered mix on hand and add your liquids as needed. Combine these ingredients and store in an airtight container, using ¾–1 teaspoon per cup of milk when ready (makes about 24 servings).

★ ¼ cup ground turmeric
★ 1 tablespoon ground cinnamon
★ 1 teaspoon ground black pepper
★ 1 tablespoon ground ginger
★ 1 tablespoon ground cloves

13. SUPERFOOD MUSHROOM HOT CACAO

Featuring a blend of herbs and mushrooms known as adaptogens, this chocolaty drink promotes a harmonious environment in the body and improves your ability to navigate stress. Each of the three key ingredients—reishi mushroom, ashwagandha root, and cacao bean—have been celebrated for centuries for their therapeutic and medicinal properties. Wrap your hands around a warm mug of comfort tonight because your hormones and sleep cycles are in for a real treat. (More good news: it doesn't taste like mushrooms.)

Reishi mushroom is called "the queen of mushrooms" for its powerful positive effects on the immune system and the gut microbiome. Ashwagandha is a popular nourishing herb that's also highly revered for its ability to soothe the nervous system and restore overall well-being. These two natural treasures can help alleviate anxiety, depression, fatigue, and insomnia. Enjoyed over a long period of time, you will notice the pleasant whole-body effect as your mental, emotional, and physical resilience is strengthened.

Whisk reishi and ashwagandha together with magnesium- and antioxidant-rich raw cacao—you won't be disappointed. The result is complete relaxation as peaceful vibes envelop you and bring you back to center. The unique combination blends seamlessly with pinches of aromatic spices, a hint of vanilla, a Medjool date or two for sweetness, and some healthy fat for absorption.

If you were scattered and restless today, allow yourself the simple, nourishing embrace that nature can offer. This gentle tonic brings patience, contentment, longevity, stamina, and stability to your whole system. Sip this warming earthy treat at least 1 hour before bedtime and allow the rest of your night to unfold naturally.

This recipe yields 1 serving.

Ingredients:

- ★ 1 cup nut milk (almond, cashew, macadamia)
- ★ 1 teaspoon organic reishi powder, or 20–30 drops extract (check brand's suggested serving size)
- ★ ½ teaspoon organic ashwagandha root powder, or 20–30 drops extract (check brand's suggested serving size)
- ★ 1 teaspoon raw organic cacao powder
- ★ Pinch ground cardamom
- ★ Pinch ground cinnamon
- ★ Pinch sea salt
- ★ 1 teaspoon vanilla extract
- ★ 1–2 Medjool dates, seeded (or 1 teaspoon raw honey)
- ★ 1 teaspoon ghee or coconut oil

Instructions:

1. Combine milk, powders, spices, salt, vanilla, and dates in a blender until smooth and creamy.
2. Heat in a small saucepan over low heat, whisking until warmed throughout and steaming, but not boiling.
3. Remove from heat and whisk in ghee or coconut oil (and honey if using) until melted and frothy.
4. Pour into your favorite mug and cuddle up for a long stress-free moment.

CHAPTER 5

RESTORATIVE YOGA POSES

Yoga is the ancient science of aligning mind, body, and spirit. The word *yoga* in Sanskrit means "union" and refers to this integration as well as the achievement of a more profound state of consciousness. As the practice encompasses not just physical postures (asanas) but also breath control (pranayama), meditation, and nutritional and behavioral guidelines, you will discover elements of yoga sprinkled throughout this book. The benefits are far-reaching and include improvements in mood, perceived stress, heart rate and blood pressure, immune and brain function, muscle relaxation, and quality of sleep. While it may not literally be the fountain of youth, it is a fountain of calm and equanimity.

A shifting perspective is perhaps the most profound gem of frequent practice. Yoga makes you teachable. Touching your toes is not as important as gaining flexibility in your mind. Synchrony of breath and movement somehow soothes the way you understand yourself and the world, opening you up to a less complicated way of living and falling asleep. Stuck or sore places suddenly become opportunities to peel away false identities and create newfound space. Positive emotions have more room to be present. You learn to make peace with yourself. In return, you build resilience to conditions like chronic stress, anxiety, depression, and insomnia.

While there are many styles of yoga, this chapter focuses on slow, passive, and supported postures that embrace comfort and simplicity. Each brings restfulness into your system and soothes stiff muscles and joints for a practice that continues to love you while you sleep. (Sitting in meditation will be more comfortable too.) Many involve resting in love for several minutes. If anything is new or you are hesitant, seek the guidance of a certified yoga instructor first.

Pair your favorite poses for a restorative sequence and perform consistently for a deeper, more restorative sleep. Practicing calm on the mat makes it easier to surrender once you're in bed. In fact, many of these poses can be performed in bed—enjoy the quiet bliss that comes, wherever you find yourself.

1. STANDING FORWARD FOLD

SANSKRIT NAME: Uttanasana (OOT-tahn-AHS-uh-nuh)
Forward folding can be incredibly healing for an overstressed mind and body. *Uttanasana* proves itself a lovely way to exit the day and enter a restorative yoga sequence—helping to relieve headaches, mild anxiety and depression, fatigue, insomnia, and built-up tension in the back, neck, shoulders, and backs of the legs. Settle into the moment as you let resistance fade away; that turns out to be a sound practice for deep sleep.

1. Begin standing tall with feet parallel, hip-width apart, hands on your hips. Inhale and lengthen your spine.
2. Exhale and fold forward from the hips, front of the torso long. Engage your core and slightly bend your knees to release tension and avoid overly rounding your upper or lower back.
3. Place your hands or fingertips on the ground or a block in front of you or beside your feet.
4. Crown of the head is heavy. Knees are bent or straight, but not locked. Hips are aligned with heels. Upper inner thighs turn slightly inward. Press heels into the floor and lift your sitting bones toward the sky, lengthening in both directions. Bring weight into the balls of your feet.
5. Rather than forcing head to knees or hands to the ground, lengthen your core and bring the belly to the thighs.
6. Inhale and extend your chest, hands down, shoulder blades gently pressing into your upper back, torso parallel to the floor. Engage your core for support. Lift your gaze forward, neck even on all four sides.

7. Exhale and melt forward, relaxing completely, neck long, quadriceps gently pressing straighter, if comfortable.

8. Breathe deeply and repeat a few times. Each inhale lengthens. Each exhale releases. With patience, your body will naturally open up.

9. Fold forward for 3 or more minutes.

10. To release, place your hands on your hips, root through your feet, engage your core, draw your tailbone down, and inhale with a flat back as you slowly return to standing.

Variations:

★ Hook the first two fingers on the big toe of each foot and wrap your thumb around your fingers, pulling up on your toes, toes pushing down into your fingers. Inhale with straight arms, exhale with bent elbows.

★ Press the palms into the calves or backs of the ankles, or tuck underneath the feet, toes meeting the wrists.

★ Sway gently side to side with bent knees, sweeping the floor with your fingertips or with hands holding opposite elbows.

★ Widen your legs for more stability. Root into the outer edges of your feet. Rest your head on a block or the ground. Hands are shoulder-width apart, elbows over your wrists and shoulder blades pressed into your back.

Do not try this pose if you have a leg, back, or knee injury.

2. CAT AND COW POSE

SANSKRIT NAME: Marjaryasana (mahr-jahr-ee-AHS-uh-nuh) and Bitilasana (bee-tee-LAHS-uh-nuh)

Though simple and gentle movements, Cat and Cow Poses together form a heart-opening sequence with powerful benefits for the mind and body. Slowly cycling through the poses stretches the abdomen, hips, shoulders, and spine while opening the chest and lungs for deep breathing. The flow improves circulation between vertebral discs and strengthens the spine, relieving pain from sciatica and menstrual cramps. Synchronizing deep breath to slow movement fosters intentional focus, emotional balance, and a calm mind—helping you shed leftover energy from the day for an easier journey into sleep.

The combination of Cat and Cow is also said to activate the second chakra, nurturing creativity and your ability to experience joy. Connect to your inner fountain of peace as you flow through this harmonizing, sleep-loving sequence.

1. Begin on a yoga mat or cushioned surface on all fours, spine flat in a tabletop position. Hips are over the knees, tops of the feet pressed into the earth. Shoulders are over the wrists, palms spread and pressed into the earth. Weight is distributed evenly through the shins and arms. Draw the navel toward your spine to engage your core, taking pressure off ankles and wrists.

2. With your gaze on the floor a few feet in front of you, roll your shoulders away from the ears, elongating your neck. Imagine the crown of your head energetically aligning with your tailbone, creating a full-body experience.

3. **COW POSE**: Inhale deeply and slowly radiate your heart forward, tailbone lifting toward the sky, belly dropping, back arching, shoulder blades spreading, head tilted with a focus on your "third eye." Gradually reach the peak of the pose with your inhale.

4. **CAT POSE**: Exhale deeply and slowly scoop the tailbone down, navel toward the spine, shoulder blades spread and rounding toward the sky, chin slowly tilting toward the chest with a focus on your nose. Gently feel the peak of the pose with your exhale.

5. Flow between Cat and Cow Poses ever so slowly, taking your time and enjoying the journey. Arms and thighs actively press into the earth, elbows straight with movement localized to the spine.

6. Continue for at least 3 minutes, coming back to a neutral spine when complete before resting in Child's Pose (see pose in this chapter).

Variations:

★ If you have wrist pain, drop down to your elbows and rest on your forearms rather than your palms.

★ If you have neck pain, keep your head in a neutral alignment with your spine without tilting.

★ If you have knee pain, place a towel underneath or fold your yoga mat for additional padding.

Do not try this pose if you have a wrist, back, knee, or neck injury.

3. CHILD'S POSE

SANSKRIT NAME: Balasana (bah-LAHS-uh-nuh)
The quintessential resting pose between yoga sequences,
Child's Pose gently stretches out the back while offering a sense
of safety and peace. Your lower back especially will thank you
for the reprieve. This mild forward bend also soothes headaches, improves blood circulation, eases tension in the chest
and shoulders, and gives the hips, thighs, and ankles a stretch.
With your forehead resting on the floor, it's as if the rest of the
world is placed on hold. The central nervous system receives
this cue to settle in for the night—it feels like a moment of
silence for your whole being.

Incorporate Child's Pose into tonight's ritual sequence and
let every ounce of stress and anxiety melt away as you sink into
a peaceful state of mind.

1. Kneel on your yoga mat, bed, or carpeted floor with the
   tops of your feet resting flat on the ground.
2. With knees and big toes touching, bring your buttocks to
   your heels and sit on your lower legs. If sitting on your heels
   is uncomfortable, place a folded blanket between your buttocks and heels.
3. Hinge at the hips and slowly fold your torso over your
   thighs. Rest your forehead on the ground in front of your
   knees, or on a blanket for more cushioning or height. Rest
   your arms along your sides, palms facing up.
4. Sink down into the earth. Melt into your hips and knees.
   Relax your shoulders away from your ears.
5. Massage your forehead with gentle back-and-forth motions.

6. Breathe fully into the back of the torso. To ease any difficulty breathing, turn your head slightly to one side.

7. Close your eyes and leave your thoughts behind while you enjoy this special space just for you and your breath. Rest here 3–5 minutes or longer.

8. To come out, press through the tailbone and use your hands to guide yourself back up. Enter an easy seated position or *savasana* to integrate the healing effects (see pose in this chapter).

Variations:

★ Separate your knees hip-distance apart, rather than joined together. Extend your arms out in front of you with palms pressed into the ground.

★ With arms in front of you, use your fingers to "walk" them to one side and then the other.

★ Widen your knees and fold your torso over a bolster or pillow, head turned to the side.

Do not try this pose if you have a knee or ankle injury, ear or eye infections, are pregnant, or have low blood pressure.

4. COBRA POSE

SANSKRIT NAME: Bhujangasana (boo-jahn-GAHS-uh-nuh)
Cobra Pose is a gentle backbend and a catalyst for transformation, improving not only posture but your capacity for giving and receiving love. Thanks to its heart-opening nature, the pose stimulates the release of endorphins, eliciting feelings of peace and joy and relieving symptoms of depression, anxiety, stress, and fatigue (which can deteriorate sleep patterns). It is also an opportunity to counteract hours spent hunched over your work and devices. With a strengthened and lengthened spine, you will feel more spacious inside and open to the gifts of sleep—less encumbered by physical and emotional pain.

1. Begin lying on your belly on a mat or cushioned surface, legs stretched back hip-width apart, tops of your feet and forehead resting on the floor.

2. Place your palms flat on the floor next to your ribs, fingers pointed forward, elbows hugged into your sides.

3. Spread your toes and gently press your feet into the earth. Engage your thighs, rotating inner thighs slightly up to broaden your lower back. Bottom and lower back are soft.

4. On an inhale, press evenly through your palms to lift your head and chest off the floor. Lower ribs and pubic bone stay on the floor. Elbows stay bent, hugged into your sides. Gaze is forward and neck is long.

5. Press your shoulder blades into your upper back to broaden your chest.

6. Do not force a deeper backbend; alignment and patience will take you much further into freedom. Instead, think about distributing the bend evenly throughout the spine.

Focus on lifting through your chest rather than pushing into your hands. Let the lift come as a natural extension of the spine.

7. As you radiate softly through your chest, make sure there is no strain on your lower back or neck. Imagine a straight line connecting feet to pelvic bone, everything touching the earth and your bottom relaxed. Shoulders drop away from your ears.

8. Breathe smoothly about 30 seconds or as long as you comfortably can.

9. On an exhale, slowly lower your chest and forehead back to the floor. Take a moment to roll your shoulders in big circles. Repeat three or more times, listening to your body.

10. To come out, engage the core and slowly push yourself up onto all fours and back to rest in Child's Pose.

Variation:

★ **SPHINX POSE**: Place your elbows on the ground underneath your shoulders, forearms extended forward. Press into the tops of your feet, elbows, and palms. Bottom is relaxed. Chin is slightly tucked with gaze forward.

Do not try this pose if you have carpal tunnel syndrome, recent back or wrist injury, or if you are pregnant.

5. SUFI GRINDING

Sufi grinds are especially popular in Kundalini yoga for their therapeutic effect on the spine and pelvic region. Both a seated yoga pose and a gentle moving meditation, Sufi Grinding involves drawing circles with your torso to evoke inner purification and reflection. Perform this relaxing exercise in the evening to open the energy of your lower spine, release tension in your back, ease stiffness in the hips, massage internal organs, aid digestion, and balance the adrenal glands. Three minutes is all it takes to feel grounded in your power and spacious inside.

To help you access your deep core of peace, recite the traditional Kundalini mantra *Sat Nam*, which can be translated as "Truth is my name." The intention is to unite breath, movement, and mantra to experience vibrational harmony with your authentic nature. What you vibrate you become, and in this way Sufi Grinding connects you to what you truly wish to manifest through your life here on earth, starting with a good night's sleep tonight.

1. Sit tall and straight in "easy pose" (legs crossed) or in a chair with your hands on your knees.

2. Close your eyes and focus on the third eye chakra (eyebrow center). Let your breathing be steady.

3. Begin rotating the lower torso in a clockwise direction, making big circles with your navel. Use slow, soft, fluid movements. Begin with smaller circles if you have low back or pelvic pain. Imagine a string lightly holding your head up. Keep your head upright and centered but allow your chin to come up naturally as you churn the spine forward.

4. Inhale deeply as you come forward over the knees and exhale as you move back. Silently repeat "Sat" on the inhale and "Nam" on the exhale.

5. As you become more comfortable, gently bring your shoulder blades together on the inhale to open the chest. As you circle back with the exhale, tuck your tummy in and stretch your shoulder blades apart to feel the stretch across your upper back.

6. After 1–3 minutes, change direction and rotate in a counterclockwise direction. Notice how this change feels and again draw your attention to the union of movement, breath, and mantra.

7. After 1–3 minutes, slowly come back to center with the spine straight for a few deep breaths. Hold a compassionate awareness of your spine.

8. Open your eyes.

To help ease constipation, Sufi Grinding can be performed for as long as 10–15 minutes in each direction. Listen to what your body needs.

Do not try this pose if you have a back or pelvic injury.

6. SEATED FORWARD FOLD

SANSKRIT NAME: Paschimottanasana
(POSH-ee-moh-tahn-AHS-uh-nuh)

This simple forward folding pose proves itself worthy of a nighttime sequence, thanks to its grounding and soothing nature. If your hips, hamstrings, back, and shoulders are tight, seated forward fold is a divine place to be. Like its standing counterpart, this pose is helpful for relieving mild anxiety and depression, headaches, indigestion, fatigue, stress, and insomnia for an overall sense of ease in the body and mind.

1. Begin seated on a mat or cushioned surface, legs together and extended straight out in front of you. Gaze is forward.

2. Rock slightly to the left and pull your right sitting bone away from the heel. Repeat on the left side.

3. Press your fingertips into the floor beside you. Root into your hips and lift upward through the spine, lengthening in both directions. Melt your upper thighs inward. Press through your heels.

4. On your inhale, raise your arms to the sky (keep on the floor if that is more comfortable).

5. Exhale as you lean forward from the hips, inching toward your feet, torso long and not rounded. Rather than focusing on how close you can get to your legs, focus on how long you can be. Think: heart toward the knee, or in the general direction of the knee.

6. Hold onto your shins, ankles, or the outer edges of your feet. If you can reach beyond your feet, clasp your wrist with your opposite hand. Bend your knees if needed.

7. Inhale and radiate your chest to find more length in the torso.

8. Exhale and, without rounding your back, release a little more fully over your legs. Let your lower belly touch your thighs first, then the upper belly, chest, and head.

9. Continue to slowly lengthen with each inhale and fold deeper with each exhale.

10. Once you are most comfortable, relax your neck and shoulders, feet and thighs slightly engaged. Soften your gaze or close your eyes.

11. Breathe here for several minutes.

12. To come out, inhale and lift the torso away from the thighs, drawing the tailbone down and engaging your core for support.

Variations:

★ Loop a strap around the soles of your feet, walking your hands down the strap as you lengthen.

★ Support yourself: Sit on a folded blanket. Rest your torso on several blankets or a pillow. Place a pillow or rolled-up blanket under your knees.

★ **HEAD-TO-KNEE POSE (JANU SIRSASANA)**: With your right leg extended, bend your left knee and rest the sole of your left foot against your right inner thigh. Fold straight over your right leg. Sink your left ribs and outer hip down. Flex both feet. Repeat on the left side.

Do not try this pose if you have recent or chronic back, hip, or ankle injuries.

7. RECLINING BOUND ANGLE POSE

SANSKRIT NAME: Supta Baddha Konasana (SOUP-tah BAH-dah cone-NAHS-uh-nuh)

Gift yourself a gentle stretch in all those areas that too often get neglected: hips, knees, inner thighs, and groin. Reclining Bound Angle Pose is a pleasant place to be if you're experiencing sciatica, back pain, menstrual discomfort, insomnia, stress, or symptoms of mild anxiety and depression. Feel the free flow of energy in your pelvis and the softening of every muscle as you check in with your body—and check out for the day.

1. Find a comfortable space on a yoga mat, carpeted floor, or in bed.

2. Roll up a blanket to the length of your entire spine and head. Place behind you and sit at one end.

3. Bring your heels toward your pelvis and let your knees fall to the sides. Give your feet a mini-massage. Clasp the soles of your feet together and sit tall.

4. Exhale and gently lower your torso onto the blanket, using your hands as support.

5. Lift your chest and draw the shoulder blades down. Lift your hips and pull your tailbone down to release the spine. Bring the heels as close to your pelvis as you comfortably can. The outer edges of your feet stay connected to the earth.

6. Imagine your outer thighs melting away from your hips and your knees falling open like wings. Imagine your inner groin sinking into your pelvis. Do not force any aspect of the stretch; let gravity work its magic.

7. Rest your arms along your sides with palms facing up. Relax your shoulders away from the ears.

8. Close your eyes and breathe easy for 5–10 minutes, or as long as you wish.

9. To come out, press your thighs together and set your feet on the floor. Lift your hips to remove the blanket from underneath you. Hug your knees into your chest and, with ankles crossed, rock side to side for a gentle massage. Roll to one side and walk yourself up with your hands into a seated position.

Variations:

★ Support the outer thighs with blankets and the knees with blocks or pillows.

★ Use a bolster or multiple folded blankets rather than a rolled blanket to support your whole back.

★ Rest only your upper back on a prop to open your chest, letting your head rest on the floor.

★ Bend your elbows at a 90-degree angle with your hands above your head (like a goal post).

Do not try this pose if you have a groin, knee, hip, or low back injury, or if you have recently given birth.

8. BRIDGE POSE

SANSKRIT NAME: Setu Bandhasana
(SET-too bahn-DAHS-uh-nuh)

A mild backbend and inversion with many different options, Bridge Pose can be both rejuvenating and luxuriously restorative. Building a strong bridge with your body—your feet and head grounded to the earth, your heart lifting toward the heavens—increases flexibility in the spine, opens the front body, strengthens the back body, and promotes stability and ease throughout. This combination soothes headaches, anxiety, backaches, menstrual discomfort, and indigestion. It's a fruitful way to "bridge the gap" between mind and body, day and night.

1. Begin lying on your back with knees bent hip-width apart, feet and toes spread evenly on the floor. Turn your heels slightly out to align with your toes. Rest your arms alongside your body, palms facing down. Tuck your chin slightly to lengthen the back of the neck. Relax your back, neck, and shoulders.

2. Walk your heels closer so you can lightly graze them with your fingertips.

3. Exhale and scoop the tailbone up, navel sinking into your spine.

4. Inhale and slowly lift your hips up, rolling the spine off the floor. Root evenly into the four corners of each foot. Gently hug your inner knees toward each other to keep the knees in line with your hips and heels.

5. Bring your shoulder blades together to interlace the fingertips beneath your bridge. Extend through the arms, pressing into the earth.

6. Gradually travel up the spine, moving your hips toward the height of your knees. Press the hips forward, not just up. Lengthen the tailbone toward the backs of your knees.

7. Firm your shoulder blades into your back to broaden and lift your chest toward your chin as your chin naturally moves away from the chest, keeping a neutral curve in the neck. Avoid turning your head to the side.

8. Stay here for 4–8 deep breaths. Watch your ribs expanding and contracting with each breath.

9. On one long exhale (or multiple breaths), slowly roll the spine to the floor.

10. Repeat, if desired.

11. When finished, hug your knees into your chest to stretch the low back. Roll to one side and walk yourself up with your hands into a seated position.

Variations:

★ Support yourself: Place a folded blanket under your shoulders. Slide a block or bolster under your sacrum and rest your hips on the support.

★ Squeeze a block between your knees for parallel alignment.

★ Externally rotate your arms so palms face the sky. Bend your elbows and rest your hands on your low back.

★ Advanced: Lift your toes and come onto the heels of your feet. Lift your arms into the air and play with fluid, circular movements, like a dance. Activate your core.

Do not try this pose if you have a neck, knee, shoulder, or back injury.

9. HAPPY BABY

SANSKRIT NAME: Ananda Balasana (AH-nun-duh bah-LAHS-uh-nuh)

A humble pose that is sure to bring a smile to your face, Happy Baby provides a gentle stretch to the hips, inner groin, and lower back, lengthens and realigns the spine, strengthens the arms and shoulders, and encourages you to view your life with childlike wonder. Its calming nature relieves stress and fatigue, making it a rather pleasant way to end today's practice—on or off the mat—and inspires a bedtime state of mind. If you go slowly and listen to your body, you'll know why *ananda* means "blissful" in Sanskrit.

1. Begin lying on your back on a thick mat, layered blankets, bed, or other cushioned surface.

2. On an exhale, hug your knees into your chest. Rock gently side to side for a few deep breaths.

3. Release your knees and keep them bent as you raise your lower legs so that the soles of your feet are facing the sky.

4. On an inhale, open your legs slightly wider than your torso and hold the outer edges of your feet, arms in front of your shins. If this feels forced, hold onto your ankles, shins, or a strap looped around the sole of each foot.

5. With shins perpendicular to the floor and ankles over the knees, pull down gently with your hands to sink the thighs closer to the floor beside you, coaxing the knees toward the armpits. Keep your feet flexed, heels extending energetically into the hands.

6. Open your chest. Relax your shoulders away from your ears by drawing them down your back. Keep the back of your neck flat, avoiding lifting the chin. Relax your head into the earth.

7. Sink the tailbone down, connecting your entire spine with the earth.

8. Close your eyes. Consciously focus on your breathing for 3 or more minutes. If it feels good, gently rock side to side for a low-back massage.

9. On an exhale, release your feet and hug your knees before rolling to your side and slowly walking yourself up with your hands.

Variations:

★ Hold on to the inside arches of your feet or hook into the big toes with your peace fingers (index and middle fingers).

★ If you have neck pain, support your head on a thickly folded blanket.

★ If you are practiced and flexible in this pose, use your hands to gently pull your legs apart, straightening the legs out to the sides for a deeper stretch.

Do not try this pose if you have a knee or ankle injury or if you are pregnant.

10. EYE OF THE NEEDLE

SANSKRIT NAME: Sucirandhrasana
(SOO-see-rahn-DRAHS-uh-nuh)

The supine version of Pigeon Pose offers a laid-back and lovely avenue for stretching the hamstrings and glutes, opening the hips, and reversing the tightness that comes from sitting for long periods of time. Eye of the Needle is thus one of the most important (and accessible) yoga poses for soothing sciatica and bringing ease into your lower half. It can even help reduce digestive discomforts and menstrual pain—further contributing to uninterrupted sleep. As your awareness naturally turns inward, physical relief isn't the only benefit you will notice: this relaxing posture is known to soothe anxiety and becalm the sea of turbulent thoughts.

1. Begin lying on your back on a comfortable, cushioned surface with your knees bent and feet flat on the floor hip-width apart. Take a few deeply calming breaths.

2. Lift your right leg, foot flexed, off the floor and cross your right ankle over your left thigh just above the knee, ankle-bone clearing your thigh.

3. Actively flex both feet to protect your ankles, pressing through your heels and pulling your toes back.

4. Use your right hand to gently press the right thigh away from you.

5. If you feel a slight pull in your right hip, stay here for several deep breaths (or for the entire length of the pose). Slide your bottom left foot farther away for a milder stretch and closer for a deeper stretch.

6. Thread your right hand between your legs and clasp both hands around your left hamstring. Use your right elbow to gently press the right knee away from you. If this is too tight, wrap a strap around your hamstring and hold the ends.

7. Lift your left foot off the earth as you bring your left leg (both feet flexed) toward the left side of your chest.

8. Keep your upper body relaxed and sinking into the earth: head, neck, shoulders. Broaden your collarbones. Tuck your chin slightly. Back is flat and hips are even on the floor. Relax your abdomen.

9. If you are limber, thread your hands even further through your legs to hold the front of your left shin. Avoid rounding your back to do so.

10. Breathe here for 3–5 minutes or longer.

11. On an exhale, release your legs and place both feet flat on the floor.

12. Repeat on the other side.

13. To come out, roll to one side and walk yourself up with your hands into a seated position.

Variation:

★ If reaching through your legs is difficult, bring your bottom leg slightly to the same side of your body. Hold your thigh with the same-side hand, and gently rest your opposite hand on your top leg's knee.

Do not try this pose if you have a knee, hip, or back injury, or if you are pregnant and past your first trimester.

11. RECLINING ABDOMINAL TWIST

SANSKRIT NAME: Jathara Parivartanasana
(JUT-ah-are-uh par-ree-VAR-tah-NAHS-uh-nuh)
Supine twists are renowned for their ability to wring out tension and stress. The gentle twisting action massages internal organs, aids digestion, lengthens the spine, stretches the hips and shoulders, and encourages deep breathing. Its naturally relaxing effects make this reclining twist a subtle yet powerful way to wind down in the evening. As you breathe stillness into your spine, breathe out energy from the day that doesn't serve you tonight.

1. Begin lying on your back on a comfortable, cushioned surface with your knees bent and feet flat on the floor hip-width apart.

2. Lengthen your back. Lift your chest and bring your shoulder blades down toward the hips, making space between your shoulders and ears. Lift your hips slightly and draw the tailbone down toward the heels.

3. Hug both of your knees into your chest.

4. With knees bent and together, exhale and use your right hand to slowly lower them over to your right side. Keep your knees above your pelvis, pointing toward your right elbow. If there is space in between your knees, fill with a folded blanket.

5. Open your arms wide at shoulder level with palms up or down. You can keep your right hand on your left knee for gentle weight. Melt your shoulders into the ground, stretching away from your ears.

6. Turn your head slightly to the left and gaze at your fingertips. You can close your eyes.

7. Hold for 3–5 minutes with smooth, steady breathing.

8. On your inhale, slowly roll your hips back to the floor, bringing your bent legs back up to center. Stay here for a moment, letting the weight of your knees sink into your low back.

9. Repeat on the left side.

10. To come out, roll to one side and walk yourself up with your hands into an easy seated position.

One-Legged Variation:

★ Hug your left knee to your chest, your right leg extended on the floor. Place your left foot on top of your right knee. Place your right hand on your left knee and slowly lower your left knee over to your right side. If there is space between your knee and the floor, slip a blanket beneath for support.

Do not try this pose if you have a recent or chronic knee, hip, or back injury, or if you have degenerative disk disease.

12. LEGS UP THE WALL

SANSKRIT NAME: Viparita Karani
(VIP-uh-REE-tuh kah-RAH-nee)

Inversions offer a beautiful spread of benefits by reversing the effects of gravity on the body. These "upside down" poses help regulate blood pressure, move stuck fluids, improve digestion, and soothe the nervous system. Legs Up the Wall is an excellent pose for relieving headaches, back pain, swollen feet, and a restless mind. Enjoy the peaceful shift in perspective as you lie down in a state of rest and surrender.

This supported variation of Legs Up the Wall uses a cushion—bolster, pillows, folded blankets—to deliver your most therapeutic experience.

1. Find an open space near a wall. Place your cushion parallel to and about 6 inches away from the wall—farther away if your hamstrings are tight and closer, even flush to the wall with a bolster, if you are flexible.

2. Sit perpendicular to the wall on the cushion.

3. With an exhale and extraordinary care, swing your legs up the wall, your head and shoulders lowering to the floor to form a 90-degree angle.

4. Once here, listen to your body. Your sitting bones drop down between the cushion and the wall—as close to the wall as is comfortable. The cushion supports the curve in your lower back. If the hamstrings are tight, bend your knees.

5. Rest your arms at your sides, palms up.

6. With legs relatively firm, slowly press the thighbones against the wall with soles facing up. Keep your legs hip-distance apart; widen for a deeper stretch.

7. Soften your throat, jaw, eyes, face, belly, and thoughts. Relax your breathing with longer exhalations. Imagine the weight of your thighbones dropping into your tailbone.

8. Rest for 5–20 minutes. If you need a break, bend the knees and bring the soles of the feet together near your pelvis.

9. To come out, slide your heels down toward your pelvis. Lift your hips to slide the prop out from underneath you; do not twist off the prop. Roll to one side and walk yourself up with your hands into a seated position.

Variations:

★ Support yourself: If your knees are bent, place a pillow behind your legs. Place a towel underneath your neck. Tie a strap around your ankles or lower legs so you can relax more fully.

★ Place a dream pillow or a cool towel with a few drops of lavender oil over your eyes. Be sure to keep your eyes closed so as not to get any oil in your eyes.

★ Hold a clear or cool-colored crystal in your hand.

Do not try this pose if you have a recent or chronic back or neck injury, glaucoma, or if you are menstruating.

13. CORPSE POSE

SANSKRIT NAME: Savasana (sha-VAHS-uh-nuh)

Savasana is considered the easiest physical pose to perform but perhaps the most difficult to master. A treat for the nervous system, *savasana* relieves stress, muscle tension, headaches, insomnia, and symptoms of anxiety and depression. You will treasure the calmer feeling state and heightened self-compassion that come with finding complete release. They are a taste of what meditation offers. It is time away from the clock. It is a place of exquisite stillness.

While learning *savasana*, keep bolsters, pillows, blankets, and a dream pillow nearby to maximize comfort and sweeten your surrender.

1. Lie down on a mat or other cushioned surface.

2. With bent knees, lift your hips and draw the tailbone down to lengthen the spine. Extend your legs and arms, ankles and hands rolling open. Snuggle your shoulder blades down your back to lift the chest. Lower your chin until your throat feels soft.

3. Close your eyes and exhale audibly several times. Return to natural breathing.

4. Invite a calm curiosity to explore the body. Notice where you make contact with the floor. Consciously soften one muscle at a time from head to toe. Exhale deeply to encourage further release. Feel your body becoming heavier, sinking into the ground, melting long-held tensions.

5. Release activity. Notice a feeling of complete stillness drawing you inward. Savor this connection with your innermost self.

6. Rest in peace for 10–20 minutes or as long as you comfortably can.

7. To come out, invite small movement into the fingers and toes. Stretch your arms over your head and rotate the wrists and ankles. Hug your knees into the chest, rolling to massage the back. Roll to one side and walk yourself up with your hands into a seated position.

Variations:

★ If you have back pain, allow bent knees to rest together; place a cushion under your knees. Alternatively, support your lower legs on a chair, couch, or bed.

★ If you have neck pain, place a blanket under your head and neck or a rolled-up towel under your neck.

★ If you have acid reflux or are pregnant, keep the head propped up with a cushion.

★ Bring your hands to your belly and breathe into your palms.

★ Breathe a mantra into each part of the body, such as "I am grounded and calm. I am melting into the earth. I am supported and safe."

Do not try this pose if you are in the third trimester of pregnancy.

Chapter 5

— **CHAPTER 6** —

MINDFUL BREATHING EXERCISES

One of the most promising strategies for calming down is also one of the simplest self-care practices: intentional breath. It is the portal to the moment lived in heightened awareness and a trustworthy companion for peaceful sleep. While fast, shallow breathing signals stress, slow, deep breathing sends a clear message that you are safe to relax—and your physiology adjusts accordingly. Each deep breath anchors you in the here and now, slows heart rate and blood pressure, melts tension and worry, and is an essential gift to your whole system. Bask in the spacious clarity that ensues because sleep naturally follows too.

Use the rituals in this chapter to free yourself from rumination and reconnect with the ancient peace you carry in your heart. To sink further into bliss, keep the following in mind:

★ Consider this a practice in gratitude and abundance. You breathe in a precious substance that is always available to you (what a gift). There is always enough for you.

★ Observe where in your body you notice your breath the most: lungs, chest, belly, back, elsewhere, everywhere. Connect with the natural rising and falling, give and take.

★ When the mind wanders, simply notice this tendency without judgment. Return to a relaxed attention on the breath. Practice compassion. Allow discomfort to dissolve into comfort.

★ If emotions come up, see them as guides. Breathe into everything. Access deeper layers of truth through the breath with curiosity.

★ Feel the connection with the formless energy your breath takes and from which all life is created and sustained. You are breathing vital life force energy (in ancient terms: *prana*, *qi*, *chi*).

★ Place handwritten cues around your home to remind you to take deep breaths.

★ Couple breath with mantra, mentally reciting phrases like "My body belongs to me. My breath belongs to me. I am here. I am powerful."

To feel fully involved with and supported by life, you may simply need to cherish this moment you're breathing in.

1. BREATH COUNTING

Breath counting is perhaps the most basic of all breathing techniques, but don't let its simplicity tempt you into dismissing its value. Keeping it simple is the best approach to cultivating a new ritual; in the case of this ritual, the beauty of simplicity is its effectiveness.

This technique helps you achieve the relaxed mental and physical state that's desirable for sleep by counting slow, rhythmic breaths. Stress is dislodged as distractions are placed on the back burner, and you will appreciate the light, centered presence you're left with. It's all about pausing to be mindful of this one moment you're breathing in and out. Doing so connects you to the silence underneath the noise—peace is a natural side effect, as is peaceful sleep.

Think of breath counting as pressing the *Refresh* button. Follow along for simply beautiful results:

1. Sit in a comfortable position with the spine straight, chin ever-so-slightly tucked. Consciously relax your limbs and muscles.

2. Close your eyes. Focus your attention on a few deep breaths, then allow the breath to come in and out naturally. Inhale presence. Exhale tension.

3. On your next exhale, silently count "one." Let your following inhale be long and full.

4. Count your next exhale as "two" and continue counting only exhalations until you reach "five."

5. Once you reach "five," begin a new cycle at "one." Do not count higher than "five." This summons a wandering mind back to the practice.

6. Continue this pattern for up to 10 minutes.

Breath counting is best learned while closing your eyes in a seated position. As you progress, you may find that you can bring this practice into other rituals. Breathe mindfully as you count to "five" before engaging in a nurturing conversation, while gazing lovingly at yourself in the mirror, or during a cooling shower. It can even make sweeping the floor a more enjoyable and enriching experience—a ritual.

MANTRA ALTERNATIVES

Try these variations, replacing numbers with five-word phrases that positively affirm your true, peaceful nature:

★ Peace. Is. My. True. Name.
★ I. Am. Loved. And. Loving.
★ Sleep. Is. My. Spiritual. Practice.
★ I. Am. Safe. And. Sound.
★ Healing. Is. Meant. For. Me.

---

2. EQUAL BREATHING

SANSKRIT NAME: Sama Vritti Pranayama
(sah-mah VRIT-tee prah-nah-YAHM-ah)

Taking an involuntary action and turning it into an intentional practice of self-nourishment is akin to transforming the mundane into a ritual. This is what you will be doing with equal breathing. In Sanskrit, *sama* means "smooth," "flat," or "same" and *vritti* means "fluctuations" or "modifications." The idea is that by focusing on equalizing the breath, you smooth the fluctuating mind. The experience can be deeply meditative, helping to pave the pathway to a deep and peaceful sleep.

No matter where you are or what you are doing, you can pause internally for one conscious breath. Equal breathing can be practiced during meal preparation, while you're listening in a conversation, as part of a walking meditation, or while you're brushing your teeth. It is simplicity at its finest. Essentially, you are remembering to breathe and that in itself is a powerful way to soothe the nervous system, repel stress, and enhance awareness. Incorporate this form of mindful nourishment into your evening routine for a touch of magic.

To feel the balancing effect of this exercise, you will breathe for equal counts through the nose, like so:

1. Inhale through the nose for a count of 4. Focus on just this one, slow, deep breath. Be fully conscious of the sensation of filling your body with nourishing air.

2. Pause for a moment (if you can) at the peak of your inhale.

3. Exhale through the nose for a count of 4, slowly and evenly. Imagine toxins and negative energies leaving your body.

4. Pause for a moment (if you can) at the emptying point of your exhale.
5. Perform as many rounds as you like.

Start with a count of 4 and adjust as needed. You can work your way up to a count of 6 or 8 as you become more practiced. Though you may feel a slight resistance at first, let this be as comfortable as possible for you, especially when you are at the beginning of creating this new pattern. If your mind wanders during breathing, be kind to yourself. Acknowledge this tendency without judgment and simply bring your mind back to one deep breath. It's all part of the practice.

3. PROGRESSIVE BREATHING

Consciously elongating your exhale by just a couple of seconds ushers your body into a parasympathetic state—slowing, soothing, and synchronizing the neural elements in your heart, lungs, and brain, which helps your body get ready for sleep. Try counting your inhale in seconds, then extend your exhale by two counts. Repeat this incredibly simple exercise to shower your entire being with healing vibrations. The benefits include relief from insomnia and anxiety, but you can practice simply for the peaceful, easy feelings.

Incorporate this breathing ritual into your nightly sleep routine and you'll find yourself dreaming in no time:

1. Begin sitting comfortably with a straight spine. You can eventually try standing, lying down, or even moving as you gain practice.

2. Close your eyes. Take a few deep inhales through your nose, exhaling out of your mouth. With each inhale, fill your lungs completely, feeling your belly expand. With each audible exhale (as if you were fogging up a window), empty yourself of air.

3. Inhale through your nose for a count of 3 seconds. Exhale through your nose for a count of 5 seconds.

4. Inhale for a count of 4. Exhale for a count of 6.

5. Inhale for a count of 5. Exhale for a count of 7.

6. Continue with this pattern—inhaling for 1 count higher than your previous inhale and exhaling for 2 seconds longer than the inhale—for as long as it is comfortable for you. Keep your breathing even and smooth.

7. When you reach your maximum capacity of inhaling and exhaling, begin moving backward. For example, if you could inhale for a count of 10 and exhale for a count of 12, your next inhale will be for a count of 9 with an exhale for a count of 11.

8. Once you reach a 3-count inhale and a 5-count exhale, release all effort. Return to normal breathing.

9. Repeat one more time, if needed.

10. Enjoy the newfound spaciousness in your mind, body, and evening.

Variations:

★ On your exhale, slightly constrict the back of your throat as if you are fogging up a window with your mouth closed.

★ Hold the breath at the top of the inhale for 1 count and do the same for the exhale.

★ Gradually build your exhale up to double the length of your inhale.

★ Repeat each same count two or three times: 3-5, 3-5; 4-6, 4-6; 5-7, 5-7; and so on.

If higher counts are too demanding, there is no need to push yourself. More important than the absolute length of your breath is that the exhale is longer than the inhale.

4. 4-7-8 BREATHING

Restful nights breed refreshed mornings, but stress has a way of hindering your ability to feel the bliss of refreshment. Practicing rhythmic breathing is like applying a soothing balm to the frazzled places within. This breathing exercise in particular is known to offer immediate relief by taming the fight-or-flight reaction, cooling your body's inflammation response and easing worried and anxious emotions. Its specific pattern—inhale to 4, hold for 7, exhale to 8—ensures that the body is receiving enough oxygen and expelling enough carbon dioxide. The balancing effect counteracts patterns of chronic stress. Ultimately, you can calm down fast and fall asleep fast, and know what it's like to wake up tomorrow feeling like your best, most rested self.

Also known as Relaxing Breath, the 4-7-8 breathing exercise positively affects blood pressure and heart rate—two systems closely linked to quality of sleep. Introduced by a Harvard-trained medical doctor as a curative for stress, anxiety, and insomnia, this supremely simple method might be just the thing you need to ease into a peaceful slumber tonight and every night.

Follow these steps to access inner calm and activate the stress-melting power of rhythmic breathing:

1. Sit comfortably with your back straight while learning this exercise. You can use a chair, the floor (with blankets and pillows as needed), or your bed to support you. Once you're familiar with the exercise, you can assume any position to practice.

2. Gently press the tip of your tongue to the roof of your mouth, just behind your upper front teeth.

3. Exhale completely through your mouth around your tongue, making a "whoosh" sound. Try pursing your lips if this feels awkward.

4. Close your mouth and inhale quietly through your nose, counting to 4.

5. Hold your breath for a count of 7 before releasing. See how soft and relaxed you can be.

6. Exhale slowly and audibly through your mouth for a count of 8, making a "whoosh" sound with your tongue in the same position.

7. Without taking a break, repeat this process three or more times.

With repetition, the 4-7-8 breathing exercise has profound effects on the body and mind. As oxygen saturates into your bloodstream, every organ, tissue, and cell is cleansed. It's a powerful way to clear your head and take care of yourself. Practice right before bedtime and through your practice, you might find that you begin to doze off within minutes, if not sooner.

If you feel lightheaded, it is usually not a cause for concern and the sensation will pass, but discontinue the practice if you are uncomfortable or strained.

5. DIAPHRAGMATIC BREATHING

Diaphragmatic breathing, also called abdominal or belly breathing, is how mammals breathe when there is no clear and present danger in their environment. We are born this way—in fact, if you watch babies breathe, you will notice their little bellies rising and falling with each breath. Shallow, chest breathing indicates perceived danger and keeps the body on high alert, leading to fatigue, anxiety, vulnerability to disease, and trouble sleeping. The slower breathing style of this exercise lets the parasympathetic nervous system take over, lowering heart rate and blood pressure, and allowing you to rest and digest.

Learn how to recruit your diaphragm so you have something familiar to return to whenever you need real rest:

1. Find a comfortable seated position: back straight, chest open, head centered. You can also lie down on a flat surface or in bed, knees bent (place a pillow or cushion underneath) and head supported. Eyes can be open or closed.

2. Consciously relax the muscles in your face, jaw, neck, shoulders, arms, and hands. Let your lips part slightly.

3. Place one hand on your upper chest and the other on your lower rib cage.

4. Inhale slowly through the nose for a count of 3–5. Feel your belly rising, rib cage expanding into your hand, your chest as still as possible. Let this feel effortless and expansive. Rather than forcing your belly out, think about your lower rib cage expanding in all directions—left, right, front, and back.

5. Notice how the peak of your inhale feels.
6. Exhale slowly and completely through your mouth for a longer or double count (ex: if you inhaled for 3 seconds, exhale for 4–6 seconds—find what is most comfortable). Feel your belly emptying, falling inward, your chest remaining still.
7. Notice the peak of your exhale.
8. Repeat this sequence for 1–5 minutes when beginning, working your way up to 10 minutes or longer.

Though simple, mastering this technique can be challenging in the beginning. For a little extra intrigue and inner exploration, play with the following variations:

★ Whisper *Haaa* during your exhale to encourage deeper relaxation.
★ Imagine you are inhaling your favorite calming scent: roses, the seaside, fresh-cut grass, a campfire, the air after a rain shower.
★ Visualize each inhale increasing pleasure-inducing chemicals in your body and each exhale sending away carbon dioxide and toxins.
★ Place both hands on your lower rib cage and focus on breathing equally into each hand.
★ Place a crystal on your chest, focusing on keeping it still.

6. ALTERNATE NOSTRIL BREATHING

SANSKRIT NAME: Nadi Shodhana Pranayama (NAH-dee SHOD-uh-nuh prah-nah-YAHM-ah)(Channel-Cleaning Breath)

In yoga, your right nostril symbolizes the energy of the sun (heating) while your left nostril symbolizes the energy of the moon (cooling). Alternate nostril breathing is a calming technique that has long been revered for its harmonizing effect on the brain and body—restoring balance to the body's opposing energies. By alternating between each nostril for the inhale and exhale, energy pathways are cleared, stray thoughts are brought back to the present moment, and the circulatory, respiratory, and nervous systems receive a healthful boost. Feeling both soothed and rejuvenated—a delicious combination—you can more easily cast aside stressful distractions and welcome bliss.

If you're feeling tense or scattered, follow this sleep-inducing sequence:

1. Sit in a comfortable position on the edge of your bed or chair with a straight spine, relaxed shoulders, and eyes closed. Breathe naturally and easily. Let your mind and body settle.

2. Place your left hand on the left knee, palm open to the sky. Press the thumb and the first finger together with light pressure.

3. Place the tips of the index finger and middle finger of the right hand in between the eyebrows, the ring finger and pinky finger near the left nostril, and the thumb near the right nostril.

4. Gently close your right nostril with your thumb and exhale slowly through the left nostril.

5. Inhale slowly and fully through the left nostril.

6. At the peak of inhalation, lightly close the left nostril with the ring finger and pinky finger. For a moment, both nostrils will be closed. Honor this brief pause.

7. Release your right nostril with your thumb and exhale slowly through the right nostril.

8. Inhale slowly and fully through the right nostril.

9. Lightly close the right nostril with your thumb.

10. Release your left nostril with your ring and pinky fingers. Exhale through the left nostril, emptying all worries from the day.

11. Inhale through the left nostril for another round, breathing in peace and harmony.

12. Continue for 3–30 minutes, starting with three to five rounds as you're learning the technique.

Feel yourself balancing and recalibrating, preparing your transition from one state of consciousness to another.

7. LEFT NOSTRIL BREATHING

SANSKRIT NAME: Chandra Bhedana Pranayama (chahn-drah BEH-dah-nah prah-nah-YAHM-ah) (Moon-Piercing Breath)

In yoga, the left nostril provides access to *Chandra* (also referred to as *Ida*) energy, which represents moon energy: cooling, soothing, yin, fluid, feminine, reflective, nurturing. Being related to the parasympathetic nervous system, spending just a few minutes breathing through the left nostril can lower your blood pressure and change your metabolism in favor of relaxation. It is a viable tool for easing anxiety, restlessness, and sleeplessness. It's almost as if the moon is lulling you to sleep from the inside out.

Prepare your body for deep and healing sleep tonight with this simple and oh-so-sweet whole-body lullaby:

1. Find a comfortable seated position, legs crossed in "easy pose," on the floor or in your bed. Spine is straight. Shoulders and jaw are relaxed. Breathe easy.

2. Rest your left hand on your thigh, palm facing toward the sky, index and thumb gently touching with the rest of your fingers relaxed.

3. Soften your gaze or close your eyes with a gentle focus on your third eye chakra (eyebrow center).

4. Gently press the right nostril closed with your right thumb, palm spreading and fingers stretched toward the sky. Imagine that your fingers are antennas for the moon's healing energy.

5. Inhale slowly through your left nostril for a count of 2–6.

6. If you are comfortable and confident in the practice, you can hold your breath at the peak of your inhale for an equal or lesser count. For example, if you inhaled for a count of 4, hold for a count of 1–4. Do not force anything.

7. Exhale through your left nostril for an equal or longer count. For example, if you inhaled for a count of 4, exhale for a count of 4–6. Slowly empty your lungs.

8. Imagine inhaling moon energy into your system. Each exhale releases tension and activity from the day. Gradually begin to feel that you are breathing in and out only soothing moon energy.

9. Continue breathing gently, evenly, and deeply in and out of your left nostril for 3–11 minutes, or longer if needed. Start with a shorter practice time and build slowly as your tolerance and confidence increases.

10. When you are finished, offer gratitude to the moon for her nurturing assistance and guidance during this practice and while you sleep.

Variation:

★ Inhale through the left nostril as usual and release the right nostril to exhale sun (or *Surya*) energy through the right nostril, gently pressing the left nostril closed with your ring and pinky fingers. Always inhale through the left nostril.

8. PURSED LIP BREATHING

Breathing is not always as easy as inhaling and exhaling. Especially for those who experience shortness of breath, breath retraining techniques such as this one can provide welcome relief and an easier entrance into sleep. Exhaling through pursed lips creates resistance in the airways, which keeps them open and allows trapped carbon dioxide to escape—saving your body from working so hard trying to force the release. This not only strengthens the lungs but also lessens the anxiety associated with difficulty breathing. A relaxed body and slower breathing rhythms are encouraged, and with them peace of mind and healthier sleep patterns.

As you practice pursed lip breathing, imagine each exhale removing stale air from your system, making room for fresh, oxygen-rich air. Inhale with gratitude. Exhale in freedom.

1. Create a peaceful atmosphere with dim lighting, slow music, calming scents, and a general sense of coziness.

2. Find a comfortable place to sit—on the floor, in a chair, or on the side of your bed. Bring in a weighted blanket or several blankets and cover your lower body to encourage a feeling of security.

3. Relax your shoulders and maintain a straight spine. To release upper body tension, roll the shoulders in a circular motion—one at a time, together, forward and backward. You may also perform a few rounds of shoulder shrugs: lift shoulders to your ears on the inhale and let them drop down on the exhale.

4. With mouth closed, inhale through your nose for a count of 2–3.
5. Pucker your lips as if you are about to whistle.
6. Exhale through pursed lips for at least twice as long as your inhale (ex: if you inhaled for a count of 2, exhale for a count of 4). Blow with the same force that you would to cool hot soup on a spoon—enough to cool, but not enough to blow it off the spoon.
7. Repeat for 3 or more minutes, or as long as you comfortably can.

Pursed lip breathing is simple in theory but may take some practice to get used to. Consider the time you spend caring for your breath as a treat for your entire being. If breathlessness sneaks into your night, you will have a familiar ritual to fall back on and regaining control over your internal landscape will become easier.

While pursed lip breathing is often recommended for patients with chronic obstructive pulmonary disease (COPD) and other respiratory conditions, it is always best to consult your medical provider before beginning a new exercise.

9. BEE BREATH

SANSKRIT NAME: Bhramari Pranayama (brah-mah-REE prah-nah-YAHM-ah)

This relaxing exercise connects breath, posture, and sound (resembling the buzzing of a bumblebee) to open the subtle energy channels of the body (also called chakras) and balance the entire nervous system. Deep vibrations soothe the spinning mind while the special hand position draws the senses inward for a complete meditative experience. The calming combination makes Bee Breath an on-the-spot remedy for mental distress stemming from anxiety, depression, and obsessive patterns. Improved concentration, headache and migraine relief, and improved quality of sleep are a few other touted benefits. Of course, you can simply practice as a way to build up your inner reserves of peace.

Follow this protocol to cut through the tangle of distracting thoughts and set your brain on the path to happiness and restful sleep:

1. Sit comfortably with your spine straight and shoulders relaxed. Lift through the crown of your head. Tuck your chin slightly.

2. With your mouth closed, keep your teeth slightly apart for the entire practice. Relax your jaw.

3. Close your eyes and concentrate on your third eye chakra (eyebrow center). Take three natural breaths through your nose.

4. *Shanmukti Mudra*: Bring your hands in front of your face with elbows pointing outward in line with your shoulders. Gently press the cartilage of your ears closed with your thumbs. Rest your index fingers above your eyebrows.

Lightly touch your middle fingers to your inner eyelids. Ring fingers rest next to the nostrils, without touching them. Pinky fingers rest on the edge of the lower lips.

5. Draw the root of the tongue to the back of the throat, creating gentle resistance so you can hear your breath.

6. Inhale naturally through your nose.

7. Exhale smoothly through your nose while making a mellow humming sound, focused at the back of the throat (rather than the front of the mouth) that resembles the buzzing of a bee or the sacred sound of *Om*. The sound continues for the whole length of your exhalation.

8. Inhale again when necessary and exhale for as long as it is comfortable. Do not force anything. Keep the shoulders and jaw relaxed. Avoid clenching the teeth.

9. Continue for several rounds—each exhale signals one round. Begin with about five rounds and gradually increase to ten rounds with practice. Imagine the vibrations connecting you to all the positive energies of the universe.

Variations:

★ As you gain confidence through practice, incorporate breath retention: inhale and hold the breath for 1–2 seconds before exhaling.

★ If this hand position feels too claustrophobic, try placing your hands on your head instead. *Helmet Mudra*: Thumbs gently press outer cartilage of the ear closed while the rest of the fingers spread along the scalp, reaching toward each other.

10. SHABAD KRIYA

A Kundalini yoga-based sleep aid, Shabad Kriya (SHAH-bhd KREE-yah) is a beautiful ritual just before bedtime or in the middle of the night to lull you back to sleep. *Kriya* refers to the union of breath, posture, and sound. Regular practice is said to significantly improve sleep duration and quality, increase intuition, balance the hemispheres of the brain, regenerate the nerves, and evoke radiance.

Shabad Kriya involves silently repeating the mantra *Sa Ta Na Ma* (Sah Tah Nah Mah), which describes the continuous cycle of life and creation; it is a wonderful catalyst for change:

★ *Sa* means "birth, infinity, totality of the cosmos"
★ *Ta* means "life, birth of form from the infinite"
★ *Na* means "death, completion"
★ *Ma* means "rebirth"

The mantra *Wahe Guru* (wah-hey goo-rro) is silently repeated on the exhale as an expression of complete ecstatic awe of the Divine; it balances the energies involved in transformation:

★ *Wahe* expresses awe and ecstasy
★ *Guru* is the one who brings us from darkness to light, from ignorance to true understanding

The elements of mantra (sacred sound), mudra (hand and eye position), and pranayama (breathing) merge into one powerful meditation that can help you break old habits, such as sleeplessness and stress, and create new positive patterns. Keep your counting slow and steady as you practice alchemy through this bedtime ritual:

1. Sit in an easy cross-legged position or in any comfortable seated posture. The spine is tall and straight. Tuck your chin slightly to open up the back of the neck.

2. Rest your hands on your lap, palms up with the right hand resting on top of the left. Thumbs tips should be touching gently and facing away from your body.

3. Softly gaze down at the tip of your nose, eyelids almost closed. Hold a relaxed awareness of the third eye (center of eyebrows). Relax your jaw and face.

4. Inhale audibly through the nose in four equal parts, mentally reciting the mantra *Sa Ta Na Ma* (one part for each "sniff"). Completely fill your lungs.

5. Holding the breath, mentally recite *Sa Ta Na Ma* four separate times for a total of sixteen beats.

6. Exhale through the nose in two equal parts, mentally reciting the mantra *Wahe Guru*. Completely empty your lungs.

7. Continue for 15 minutes (or for as long as you can) and up to 62 minutes, and any amount of time in between.

8. To end, take a breath in and out normally. Bring your palms together in front of you (as if you are praying or saying "namaste" at the end of a yoga practice) and chant, sing, or speak one elongated *Sat Nam* (the "seed" mantra of *Sa Ta Na Ma*).

To establish restorative sleep rhythms, practice Shabad Kriya several nights a week or in a row.

11. UJJAYI BREATHING

Ujjayi (oo-jai-ee) is an ancient yogic breathing technique commonly referred to as the "oceanic breath" due to the specific sounds that are created through the breath, which resemble waves crashing into the shore. This is a wonderful practice for connecting with your inner guidance system and letting it lead you into the realm of sleep. Ujjayi breath will center your focus and soothe the psyche, removing anything distracting you from a good healing slumber.

When feelings of agitation or stress are lingering from the day, try this balancing sequence to regain your power and find your center—because you are as vast as the sea:

1. Find a comfortable seated position, either in a chair, cross-legged, in lotus pose, or any other position that feels good to you. Keep your back straight, hands resting on the knees with palms facing upward. Close your eyes and exhale completely, sending out all of the energy of the day.

2. Seal your lips and breathe in and out through your nose several times, until you feel you have an easy, fluid rhythm. Let your breathing be as natural as the rolling tide.

3. Take a deep, steady breath in through your nose, mindfully inhaling through both nostrils evenly. Fill yourself completely. Let your belly extend outward, grateful for receiving this breath. Each inhale is like water gathering up to form a wave.

4. Pause at the peak of your inhale—the crest of the wave—for a moment to bask in the fullness of your breath.

5. Exhale slowly and deeply through your nose, completely emptying your lungs. While exhaling, pull your abdominal area back to the spine. Feel the passage of outgoing air on the roof of your mouth. The sighing sound your breath makes is similar to the "*Haaa*" sound you make when you're fogging up a window, except that your mouth is closed. Compare this sighing sound to a wave crashing.

6. Pause for a moment to feel the spaciousness inside of you before you begin another round of inhaling through the nose.

Each exhale signifies the wave crashing into shore. Repeat for a minimum of five rounds and, as your practice grows, progress to up to 10 minutes of Ujjayi breathing. To unite your practice with the restful sleep that is ahead of you, lie down in *savasana* (see Chapter 5) on the ground or in your bed.

12. RAINBOW BREATHING

As the name implies, this breathing exercise involves focusing on the seven colors of the rainbow. You will naturally be prompted to visualize each color as you "breathe it" in and out. Rainbow breathing creates a sense of harmony and energetic balance within the body while giving the mind something easy to focus on other than what happened today or ten years ago, or what might or might not happen tomorrow. Practice when you need an easy way to conjure up bedtime vibes in *this moment*. A soothing experience in the bathtub or while brewing tea, it is readily accessible and can be used alongside many other rituals for an altogether magical experience—the rainbow is one of nature's most beautiful phenomena, after all.

As you breathe through the colors, imagine breathing in each color's energetic qualities, which are in the following list for guidance. Stay with each color for as long as you like, paying attention to what color is drawing your attention and asking for more time. Listen to your body's response and sense the subtleties of the messages that come up. Of course, you can simply use this exercise as a quick way to interrupt stressful thoughts and focus on your breathing so you can get to bed easier tonight.

For each color, you will:

1. Breathe in for a count of 4.
2. Hold for a count of 1, if you comfortably can.
3. Breathe out for a count of 4.
4. Hold for a count of 1, if you comfortably can.

5. Repeat two more times for a total of three rounds before moving to the next color.

As you become more practiced and relaxed in your rhythmic breathing, you can progress to a count of 6 then 8 on the inhale and exhale. Let your breathing be easy at all times. Repeat for more than three rounds for any colors that feel particularly good to breathe in.

Begin with red and move your way to violet, focusing on the energy and qualities of the color:

1. **RED**: Passion. Vitality. Comfort. Security. Safety.
2. **ORANGE**: Warmth. Creativity. Playfulness. Trust. Core desires you would like to manifest.
3. **YELLOW**: Joy. Clarity. Patience. Acceptance. Healing light.
4. **GREEN**: Growth. Fertility. Balance. Wealth. Good health. Compassion. Love.
5. **BLUE**: Peace. Understanding. Hope. Optimism. Embrace of the unknown.
6. **INDIGO**: Serenity. Self-awareness. Intuition. Deep peace. Divinity.
7. **VIOLET**: Appreciation. Highest self. Consciousness. Freedom. Transcendence. Enlightenment.

Imagine that every cell is bathing in the vibrant, colorful oxygen you're breathing in. You might even imagine a beautiful spectrum of light inside as you are graced with the healing properties of each color.

CHAPTER 7

MEDITATIONS FOR DEEP RELAXATION

Meditation is the practice of remembering who you are and who you are not, of being intimate with life as it is. Rather than being perfect, meditation is simply about showing up for whatever arises in the moment—thoughts, emotions, stories, sensations—and recognizing that you are not what you're witnessing because *you are the witness*. Seeing your patterns in this way disarms habitual storylines and restores your power to compose an experience that's more favorable to sleep.

Regular practice inspires measurably positive changes associated with sense of self, stress, mood, memory, information processing, and focus. Aside from cultivating a stronger sense of peacefulness in your mind and body, meditating in the evening gives you a chance to reinterpret the day—and yourself—through the lens of compassion. The perspective shift turns mistakes and heartaches into guides instead of chains. Redirecting feels like sweet relief. With a slower heart rate and lower blood pressure, breathing yourself to sleep becomes more and more of a reality.

The goal here is not to magically empty your mind and erase emotions but rather to witness them with non-judgmental awareness for nanoseconds at a time. When you get distracted by the natural wanderings of your mind, start again. Then, stay open to whatever intelligence arises.

You may choose to create a designated space with soothing sights, scents, sounds, blankets, and cushions to support your practice. For small spaces, you can set up an altar on a table, keep tools like a notebook and incense inside a drawer, or hang a vision board with pinned mantras and poetry. You can sit or lie down, you can use an object or a phrase as a focal point or not, you can practice for 1 minute or 20 minutes—however you choose to meditate, remember that there is no such thing as a wrong way.

The meditations in this chapter are designed to let sleep come to you. They are not strict formulas but invitations to explore the rest between breaths and the stillness underneath the chatter. Come as you are and be as you are because this is *your* practice.

1. MINDFULNESS MEDITATION

Mindfulness is the subtle art of keeping yourself company. It requires intimacy with the present moment, turning it into a complete sensory experience. Doing so can break the chain of stress, worry, and rumination; improve memory, concentration, and decision-making; improve overall physical health; and disarm thoughts that hinder a peaceful slumber. Stay a few heartbeats longer and you will get to feel your life as you live it.

Leave room for wonder and curiosity because these are necessities for serendipity: finding something meaningful in an unexpected place, like the present moment. You will deepen your connection to the sights and sounds of nighttime, which shows kinship with sleep. Also, don't worry about not doing this "right." Mindfulness isn't about erasing thoughts, emotions, or sensations but developing a more compassionate relationship with them. Observing the tendencies of the mind and consciously redirecting it to the moment are part of the practice.

1. Find a comfortable place to sit for 5–10 minutes or more— back straight, palms on thighs.

2. Breathe easily through your nose. Each breath takes you deeper into the moment and a receptive nature.

3. Set an intention to stay in an open awareness that takes note of every sensation. Let any thoughts that arise come and go without judgment. Gently return your awareness to your breathing and senses as often as needed.

4. Focus on what you see: every edge, curve, color, pattern, size, or movement. Experiment with narrowing your gaze to

one object, and then expanding it to take in more of your environment.

5. Focus on what you hear: your own breathing and heartbeat, soft or loud noises, voices, the silence underneath it all.

6. Focus on what you can smell: fresh flowers, what's baking, essential oils diffusing, the lotion on your skin.

7. Focus on what you feel: every texture, subtle movement, what's supporting your body, the clothing on your skin, how the air feels, your lungs filling and emptying, where your hands are resting.

8. Focus on any tastes you can detect in your mouth. If you cannot, notice this too.

9. Observe the interplay of all five senses. Contemplate this moment as if you are creating a memory. Savor this moment without needing it to be any different than it is.

10. When complete, allow yourself to bask in the comfort and tranquility of your own acceptance of the present moment. Come back to this mindful awareness anytime—even for 10 seconds at a time.

You can sit quietly or bring mindfulness to any activity, such as washing the dishes. Practice maintaining an awareness of a particular object while also holding a wider awareness of your surroundings—for example, perceiving the whole room while also seeing the details of the dish.

2. COMPASSIONATE BODY AWARENESS

Consider this: you are here in physical form because the universe longs to experience itself through you. A regular practice of self-compassion is an expression of gratitude for this miracle called life, however it happens to appear. Performing a body scan with this compassionate awareness can prove to be much more than a way to soothe the mind—it is a ministry of presence. This approach both balances the tendency to "live in your head" and develops a more helpful relationship with yourself that allows for inner peace. Over time, you can explore emotions in a non-judgmental way. Your progression toward greater unity between the body and self is an open invitation for a night of real rest.

The goal of this meditation is not to force a feeling, but to simply feel. A ministry of presence is a practice of leaning in and allowing. Even drifting thoughts are part of the meditation. Use this practice to bring a quality of spaciousness into your evening and to soften the pangs of insomnia and inner criticism.

1. Lie down comfortably on a cushioned surface or bed and sink into this support. Close your eyes.

2. Place your hand on your heart and feel it beating, sending your body the message that it's safe to relax.

3. Place your other hand on your belly, feeling it rise with each inhalation. Observe the breath. Notice how it feels to be in your body, lying on this surface, breathing this air.

4. Release your focus on the breath and invite a friendly curiosity into your left big toe. Just observe and let it be felt. Move your focus to your other toes, heel, and bottom of the foot.

Hold a compassionate awareness no matter what sensation arises—tension, sadness, boredom, even the absence of feeling.

5. Attend to the whole body in this same way—right foot, legs, hips, bottom, belly, back, hands, arms, shoulders, chest, neck, face, and head. Spend about 1 minute with each area. If the mind wanders, simply notice that too. Loosen your attachment to any unhelpful phrases or unwanted emotions that come up, letting everything come and go. Drift back to a kind curiosity of your physical body. Lean into the subtle nuance of sensation with acceptance.

6. Once every area has received this awareness, widen your awareness and let it drape over your entire body.

7. Rest here for several breaths.

8. When ready, come back to your awareness of your hands on your belly and on your heart. Open your eyes and stretch gently.

As you nestle into bed, loosely contemplate how amazing it is that you have a body to experience life through.

3. LOVINGKINDNESS (METTA) MEDITATION

Metta is the unconditional lovingkindness of the universe. The idea of this practice is to become a channel for universal love—the vital currency and essential foundation of all life. As you breathe metta (lovingkindness) in and out, you will observe how every single grievance and frustration from the day fades away. This meditation will quickly take you from feelings of "less than" or blame or separation to an overwhelming sense of wholeness and fulfillment. Its ability to inspire harmony makes metta the perfect ingredient for a restorative night's sleep.

If judgment rests in your heart, apply this lovingkindness meditation as you would a healing salve. Practice each step for 1 minute or as long as needed before moving on to the next:

1. Sit comfortably. Place your left hand on your heart. Let your right hand fall relaxed at your side or on your lap, palm facing upward. Close your eyes and breathe easily. Imagine the breath moving through the area of your heart.

2. Invite any grievances to come and be resolved. Let them rest in your awareness.

3. Now, breathe in the unconditional lovingkindness of the universe. Let it fill your heart with compassion and then breathe out any tension and frustration. With each inhale, feel this metta expand to a universal acceptance and forgiveness. With each exhale, you empty yourself of stress.

4. When you are feeling more spacious inside, breathe in lovingkindness and let it flood your whole body, toe to crown. Breathe it back out into the world.

5. Breathe in metta and breathe it out, letting it flow now to your loved ones. Imagine this energy flowing into their hearts too.

6. Breathe in, letting metta fill every cell in your body, and breathe it out, sending it now to anyone with whom you have a grievance. You are simply breathing out what you have received. Let your heart stay open to this exchange of source energy.

7. Breathe in sweet metta, and feel it ripple through you. Let it flow out to every sentient being on the planet, protecting everything with love and light.

8. Breathe in again and radiate this healing energy into every corner of the galaxy.

9. Take a big inhale and feel universal love energy rushing back to you. Breathe it back out into the world.

10. Return to regular breathing. Sense barriers fading. See how precious all forms are and how giving and forgiving the formless is. Sit here for as long as you like.

When there is only love flowing through you, there is no room for anything that is not love. Notice now how you are a conduit for universal love. Fall asleep with your hand on your heart if you need to reconnect.

4. CANDLE GAZING MEDITATION

Known as *Trataka* in Sanskrit, meaning "to gaze," this open-eye meditation combines the entrancing qualities of fire with focused awareness. By fixing your gaze on the flickering flame of a candle, the wavering mind stills and opens to peace. It is said to provide deep relaxation, enhance memory and concentration, improve eyesight, strengthen intuition, and stimulate the pineal gland—an endocrine organ in the brain that produces melatonin and is often referred to as the "third eye."

Give yourself some much-needed mental space with this enchanting meditation:

1. Create a dimly lit space that is free from clutter.
2. Set up a comfortable place to sit, on a cushion or in a chair with feet flat on the floor.
3. Place your candle in front of you on a flat surface, at eye level, 1–3 feet away. Ensure there are no cross-breezes or flammable items nearby.
4. Envision the qualities you would like to bring into your night (peace, protection, and so on) and light the candle. Believe in the magic of the fire to support your desires.
5. Breathe softly and easily through your nose as you settle down. Keep your spine straight and upright.
6. With a soft gaze, focus on the candle's flame. Let all other movement and thought be still. If your eyes begin to water, close your eyes and focus on your third eye (center of the eyebrows). Let the image of the candle fill your mind.
7. When your mind wanders, gently return to the flame and your breathing. Repeat.

8. Imagine breathing the light energy inside of you, filling you with the qualities you need for a restful sleep. Exhale as this energy bathes you in light.

9. Continue for 3–5 minutes while learning, gradually increasing practice time.

10. As your meditation draws to a close, close your eyes for a few rounds of deep breathing.

11. Extinguish the flame with gratitude. Imagine the smoke carrying your intentions into the invisible realm from which creation and dreams arise.

12. Lie down in *savasana* (see Chapter 5) or in bed with eyes closed, focusing on the flame in your mind's eye. Enjoy the sweetness of centered focus and the sweet slumber that follows.

CANDLE MEANINGS

Choose 100 percent soy, beeswax, or ghee candles that are free from chemicals. (Crystal or Himalayan salt tea light versions bring their own healing properties.) Coordinate color with your intentions to elevate your practice:

★ White: Peace. Divination. Healing.

★ Violet: Spirituality. Intuition. Psychic abilities.

★ Indigo: Wisdom. Truth. Self-awareness.

★ Green: Love. Fertility. Abundance. Health.

★ Pink: Nurturing. Compassion. Calms emotions.

★ Yellow: Joy. Banishes depression.

★ Orange: Creativity. Resilience. Attraction.

★ Brown: Grounding. Stability.

★ Black: Protection. Dispels negative energy.

5. HIMALAYAN SALT LAMP MEDITATION

When the sun sets, sleepy energy is supposed to settle in. Basking in the blue light of your devices muddles with this natural process by tricking the brain into thinking that it is still daytime. Meditating on the gentle orange hues of a Himalayan salt lamp brings the energy of the setting sun to you. Not only a helpful focal point for meditation, this environmentally-friendly light source diffuses negative ions that can help purify the air, neutralize electromagnetic radiation, improve mood, and elicit deep sleep.

Relax into a peaceful state of mind, courtesy of your salt lamp's hypnotic glow:

1. Create a comfortable atmosphere around your salt lamp where you will not be disturbed. Remove all devices. Play nature-inspired music.

2. Find a comfortable seated position in front of your lamp on a blanket or pillow, one leg crossed in front of the other or in a chair or bed with feet flat on the floor. Root into the earth. Lengthen your spine. Soften your shoulders and face. Relax your breathing.

3. Begin acquainting yourself with your lamp. Touch and admire its texture, shape, edges, hues, and warmth with an open curiosity. Bask in its gentle energy.

4. Rest your hands on your thighs for a few breaths, infusing them with warm positive energy. Spine is long. Your gaze rests on the lamp.

5. On a long inhale, bring your hands to your sides, palms up, and slowly raise your arms overhead from the sides as if you were scooping all the energy of the earth up into the sky.

6. Exhaling, bring your hands back down in front of you, palms facing you, as if you were showering yourself in the earth's healing energy.

7. Continue synchronizing your breathing to movement for 3–11 minutes. Gaze at the lamp—eyes open or closed, seeing the lamp in your mind's eye.

8. Each inhale gathers warm positive energy from your salt lamp, melting thoughts and tension. Each exhale showers you in healing light. Inhale to receive. Exhale to bathe.

9. When you feel you are finished, inhale deeply and stretch your arms up over your head. The palms meet.

10. On your exhale, slowly bring your hands, palms together, down in front of your heart. Thumbs press into your chest, fingers spreading.

11. Eyes closed, thank your salt lamp for removing impurities and summoning sleep.

12. Rest here for a few deep breaths. Open your eyes. Imagine the glow of the lamp comforting you through the rest of the night.

To remind you of the peace that you felt during this meditation—and to encourage sleepy energy to flood your brain and body—keep a Himalayan salt lamp in your bedroom (or in every room).

6. HEALING CRYSTAL MEDITATION

Formed deep in the heart of the earth, crystals have been used for thousands of years to heal the mind, body, and soul. Each natural formation is believed to harness unique healing qualities that work to amplify intentions and address imbalances. Meditating with sleep-supporting crystals provides a sense of well-being and nudges you in the direction of restoration. If you are new to the concept of using crystals, open your heart to the subtle life energy flowing through all things. An open heart will take you into a deeper meditation for easier sleep.

Select your crystal based on a specific intention or need. If you feel drawn to a particular crystal, follow that intuitive guidance. There are several that can help you unwind before bed:

★ **CLEAR QUARTZ**: "Master healer." Pure positive energy. Balancing. Enlightenment.

★ **SELENITE**: Alignment with highest potential. Mental clarity. Relieves stagnation.

★ **HOWLITE**: Sleeping aid. Dream retention. Stress relief. Dissolves pain.

★ **MOONSTONE**: Divine feminine energy. Inner wisdom. Patience. Infinite possibilities. Enhances intuition.

★ **CELESTITE**: Universal wisdom. Restful sleep. Renewed hope. Angelic protection.

★ **AMETHYST**: Releases negativity and anxiety. Soothes trauma. Inner guidance.

★ **LAPIS LAZULI**: Spiritual journeying. Dream work. Destiny.

★ **APOPHYLLITE**: Soothes fears and frayed nerves. Angelic connection. Courage and authenticity. Contentment.

★ **ROSE QUARTZ OR RHODONITE**: Eternal, unconditional love. Forgiveness. Emotional healing.

★ **TURQUOISE**: Protection. Spiritual balm for old emotional wounds and chronic stress. Health and abundance.

★ **SMOKY QUARTZ**: Grounds and balances. Protects from nightmares. Absorbs and transmutes negative energy, painful memories, and electromagnetic radiation.

To clear your crystal of old or unwanted energy:

★ Envelop it in sage or Palo Santo smoke

★ Lay it on a piece of selenite or clear quartz for a few hours

★ Place it under full moonlight for a few hours

★ Place it in the soil or amongst the leaves of a healthy houseplant overnight

★ Bury it in the earth overnight

Once cleansed, begin your meditation:

1. Find a comfortable seated or lying down position.

2. Hold your crystal. Imagine that your crystal is downloading your intentions.

3. With a clear mental image of your crystal, close your eyes. Pause for a few deep breaths to solidify your connection.

4. Continue holding your crystal or place it on the area of your body where you most need relief or strength. Feel its weight.

5. Envision breathing your request "into" the crystal and inhaling the crystal's healing energy in return. Sense its vibrational qualities filling you, answering your requests with the essence of your intentions.

6. Move back and forth between an awareness of your breath and your crystal.
7. When you are ready, slowly transition back to your evening with this awareness.
8. Place the crystal on your nightstand, under the foot of your bed for grounding, or under your pillow to lull you into a deep slumber.

7. MALA MEDITATION

Traditionally a string of 108 beads, a mala is used to count a mantra—a sacred sound or intention—during meditation. Aside from the 108 counting beads, the garland features a larger symbolic "guru bead" and a tassel where all threads unite. Using a mala is similar to using a rosary in that it brings a tangible element to your practice. It can help slow respiration, keep you focused and grounded, encourage a sense of well-being, and connect you to a deeper understanding of yourself. This makes the mala a powerful tool on your journey inward toward peace and peaceful sleep.

Mantras are carefully chosen phrases carrying a specific energetic vibration meant to still the mind. Here are some options in Sanskrit, a language designed to reach the depths of your being:

★ *Om* (Aum or Ohm): The vibration of the universe.

★ *Shanti* (Shahnti): Peace.

★ *So Hum*: "I am That," meaning "I am that which is infinite and eternal."

★ *Sa Ta Na Ma* (Sah Tah Nah Mah): Powerful change.

Consider what qualities you would like to invite and listen to what sounds and feels right for you. Create a phrase using your native language if that's more comfortable—such as "I am enough" or "I radiate peace." Remember: This is *your* practice.

Follow these steps to begin your journey into a state of consciousness that coincides with sleep:

1. Find a comfortable seated position. Rest your mala easily over the ring finger of your dominant hand. Settle in and close your eyes.

2. Start with the first bead after the guru bead. Repeat your mantra out loud.

3. Use your thumb to gently pull each bead over the finger toward you, reciting your mantra with each bead. Synchronize your breath with the action.

4. As you continue, begin to whisper and then silently recite your mantra, bringing your practice inward.

5. When you reach the guru bead, do not count or pass over. Take this moment to offer gratitude for a teacher, healer, spiritual guide, or your inner guide.

6. Flip the mala over and work your way back or stop here for a quiet moment before ending your practice. Absorb your mantra, letting it flow over you. Slowly continue with your evening.

Choosing a mala is as personal as your practice. Malas can be made from wood, seeds, or crystals, each with their own healing properties. Trust your intuition to guide you to the materials that resonate with you. When not in use, treat your mala respectfully: place it carefully in a wooden box or pouch for safekeeping or drape it lovingly on an altar or near a plant. Include it in a cleansing ceremony whenever you'd like to clear its energy and start anew.

8. CHAKRA HARMONY MEDITATION

Chakras are concentrated centers or "wheels" of energy within the body where vital life force energy flows. A chakra that is open and "spinning" propels optimal health on all levels—physical, mental, emotional, spiritual—whereas a blocked chakra is believed to manifest issues in the body and in life. This self-balancing meditation opens and aligns the chakras so that energy flows freely in all directions, dissolving stress and promoting rest.

Consult the following seven major chakras with corresponding colors, mantras, and crystals to help restore harmony and summon sleep:

1. **ROOT CHAKRA**: Base of the spine. Denotes stability, safety, fearlessness. Color: red. Crystal: red jasper, obsidian, garnet. Mantra: Lam, "I am safe."

2. **SACRAL CHAKRA**: Below the navel. Denotes abundance, pleasure, well-being, sexuality. Color: orange. Crystal: moonstone, carnelian, tiger's eye. Mantra: Vam, "I am creative."

3. **SOLAR PLEXUS**: Upper abdomen. Denotes vitality, self-worth, self-confidence, empowerment. Color: yellow. Crystal: citrine, golden calcite, yellow fluorite. Mantra: Ram, "I am strong."

4. **HEART CHAKRA**: Just above the heart. Denotes love, empathy, forgiveness, trust. Color: green. Crystal: jade, rose quartz, malachite. Mantra: Yam, "I am loved."

5. **THROAT CHAKRA**: Throat. Denotes self-expression, truth, communication. Color: blue. Crystal: aquamarine, sodalite, turquoise. Mantra: Ham, "I am expressive."

6. **THIRD EYE CHAKRA**: Eyebrow center. Denotes intuition, imagination, concentration, wisdom. Color: indigo. Crystal: amethyst, lapis lazuli, apophyllite. Mantra: Sham, "I am connected."

7. **CROWN CHAKRA**: Top of the head. Denotes connection to spirituality, higher purpose, pure bliss, devotion, enlightenment. Color: white, violet. Crystal: clear quartz, selenite, howlite. Mantra: Om, "I am divine."

Use this meditation to paint harmony within the physical and energetic body:

1. Settle into a comfortable seated position, cross-legged or on the edge of a chair or bed with your spine straight.

2. Beginning with the root chakra, touch your hand or associated crystal to your skin where the chakra is located.

3. Close your eyes and consciously breathe into and from this space.

4. Visualize the colored light swirling in a clockwise motion, healing issues and removing blockages. Recite your mantra silently.

5. Move up into the next chakra when it feels right. Work your way up through each chakra in the same way.

6. Once you've "opened" your crown chakra, visualize white light streaming down through each energy center, one by one turning the colors bright and clear.

7. Sense the integration of the spinning chakras as light flows effortlessly up and down your spine, showering you with good health.

8. Inhale energy rising toward liberation. Exhale energy descending toward manifestation.
9. When your practice feels complete, imagine each chakra from crown to root closing like a flower at night.

Now you can prepare for sleep feeling grounded, emotionally strong, and connected to your higher self—whole and harmonized from head to toe.

9. YOGA NIDRA

Literally meaning "yogic sleep," this whole-body therapy introduces you to a dreamy state between waking and sleeping—1 hour might be as effective as 3 hours of regular sleep. With roots going back thousands of years, Yoga Nidra has revealed its profound potential to heal psychological wounds, emotional trauma, addiction, anxiety, depression, insomnia, and chronic tension. More immediate benefits include reduced stress and better sleep. Perhaps it is the forgiving nature of the practice that engenders a sense of union with the entire universe—dissolving the painful illusion of separateness.

Use this script to melt into the peace that runs deeper than any disturbance, taking several minutes with each step, if you can:

1. Lie down on your back (see *savasana*, Chapter 5) in a peaceful environment and be as comfortable and cozy as possible. Use a dream pillow or simply close your eyes.

2. Bring to mind your heartfelt desire or intention for this practice: to relax deeply, support sleep, induce healing, etc. Then, let it go. The essence of your intention remains even after you consciously release it.

3. Invite an open curiosity of your surroundings. Welcome all sounds, smells, tastes, and sensations with acceptance.

4. Become aware of your breathing, in and out the nose. Notice how each exhale releases a bit of tension and each inhale fills you with new oxygen.

5. Envision an internal safe haven, a place you can return to if a particularly distressing sensation comes up—you can place your hand on your heart if that resonates.

6. Scan your body, gradually moving through one muscle, bone, organ, and region at a time: scalp, forehead, eyes, nose, ears, jaw, inside the throat, and so on, all the way to your toes. Welcome whatever you find without needing to change anything.

7. Let your awareness rest over your entire body. Observe and welcome any surfacing emotions and thoughts with calm attention.

8. Sense an unchanging peace underneath what is always changing, a stillness that runs deeper. Sense the space in between your cells.

9. Feel your body breathing effortlessly like it is asleep. Pay attention to the emptiness at the end of your exhale, and how the next breath arises from that. Notice the same stillness at the peak of your inhale and how it sparks the next exhale.

10. Every "I am" dissolves in this deep pool of well-being.

11. Reconnect with your desire. Feel it emanating from the silence between breaths, the space between cells, flowing from the unchanging foundation of all life.

12. Reorient to your surroundings, honoring the quiet stillness from which every sound and activity is born.

13. Bring gentle movement into your fingers and toes. Breathe gratitude for taking this time to be still. Open your eyes when ready.

10. NATURE WALKING MEDITATION

Being in mindful contact with nature is a powerful reminder that beauty is everywhere—shining forth from every little flower and patient tree, from the light dancing on the water's surface, from the celestial celebration in the night sky. As you witness the majesty of the setting sun and budding stars with renewed wonder, you may find peace easier to come by tonight.

A regular nature walking meditation offers a chance to interact with the abundant beauty and healthful benefits of the earth. Natural sights and sounds are intrinsically calming. Pondering the variety of life encourages a shift in perspective. Even a short amount of time in nature each evening can help you heal your mind and body: lowering stress, improving mood, slowing heart rate, normalizing blood pressure and respiration, improving sleep rhythms, and bridging the gap between you and everything around you.

Let your body intuitively guide you along your chosen path through scenery you enjoy. Move at a slow pace that reserves space for reflection and pure awareness. Wear layers if it's a cooler season, and bring a blanket or mat if you choose to take a sitting break. You can share this time with a loved one, agreeing to walk together in silence and joy.

Treat the following suggestions as loose guidelines from which you can build a mindful, self-guided tour in any way that feels most natural to you:

★ Appreciate every pebble, leaf, blossom, and animal you pass by. Offer the blessing of your full presence.

★ Let nature effortlessly enter through all your senses. Look at the big and little details. Listen to the critters and breeze.

Smell the fragrances. Feel your own movement. Drink in the flavor of your surroundings.

★ Practice *earthing* by making direct physical contact with the earth through your bare skin. Place your hands on a tree. Caress the petals. Dip your fingers or toes in the stream. Walk barefoot in the dirt or grass, if you can. Feel recharged through the energy source of the planet.

★ Be humbled, surrounded by so much vitality, creativity, and intelligence. Be honored, knowing that you are part of everything you notice. As you look at nature with love, you may find it easier to look at yourself with love.

★ If your mind wanders from your present-moment experience, just return to a restful, open awareness. Every step and return to nature is a celebration of your profound and unfathomable connection.

★ If you wish, spread out your blanket or mat, pausing for a moment of stillness. Otherwise, continue to walk back home.

Carry this deep resonance to bed. Thank the earth for providing you with all the energy you need to live, breathe, and dream.

11. HEALING HANDS

Our hands express what is known in Hindu philosophy as *prana*, the "life force" or "vital principle" comprising all the light, love, and energy of the universe. In this meditation, you activate your hands to be an even greater source of healing—for you and for everyone and everything around you. You can engage the practice to invoke and impart peaceful blessings as you set up your physical space and headspace for more harmonious sleep rhythms.

Adapted from a Kundalini yoga method, this practice directs the flow of energy through your hands using your conscious awareness. By magnifying this vital energy, you will feel as though you're vibrating in unison with the whole universe. You will radiate the kind of deeply calming energy that invites sleep and your touch will be soothing to all who receive it (including yourself).

The ritual takes about 11 minutes. Follow along to deliver a touch of grace to your night:

1. Find a comfortable seated position and close your eyes.
2. Gently rub your palms together for 3 minutes, focusing on the sensation and heat generated between your hands. Breathe naturally.
3. Stretch your arms out to the sides of your body at shoulder height, parallel to the floor with palms facing up and thumbs pointing behind you. Keep your elbows soft, not locked or forced.
4. Take long, deep breaths in and out through your nose, mouth closed, your diaphragm extending on the inhale and

contracting on the exhale. Visualize your hands receiving all the light, love, and energy of the universe. Stay here for 3 minutes.

5. At the top of your inhale, hold your breath gently. Turn your wrists so that your palms are facing away from your body, as if you're pushing against the walls on either side of you.

6. Exhale audibly and send your breath into the center of your palms.

7. Inhale and imagine all the cosmic energy you've received condensing, absorbed into the center of your palms.

8. Breathe like this for another minute or so. Feel the light from your hands beginning to flood your entire body.

9. Exhale and move your hands in front of you, elbows bent and forearms parallel to the floor, so that your left palm is in front of your stomach facing up and your right palm is in front of your chest facing down. Feel the magnetic force of the energy exchange between your palms. Stay here for 3 minutes.

10. Release your position and continue with your evening, mindful of the energy you carry.

Practice immediately before other rituals for a more intimate and powerful experience. For instance, you could use this in conjunction with a self-message, when handling sacred objects or food, or while interacting with loved ones.

12. PONDERING INSPIRATIONAL TEXT

There is something soul-soothing about holding a book in your hands after a long day in a busy digital world, especially when you're returning to the quiet comfort of something you love. Reading lowers stress, eases symptoms of depression, enhances imagination, improves memory and focus, brightens the mind, and tires the eyes—putting you in the right frame of mind for sleep. Even better is if what you're reading inspires you to fall asleep with wonder in your heart.

If you are used to rushing through pages, note that this is a different kind of reading. As you move slowly and contemplatively, you become more mindful of the moment and the energy coming through the words. Take your time and rest in stillness (that's what nighttime is for).

Explore what inspires your mind, opens your heart, and soothes your soul tonight:

★ **FICTION NOVELS**: Leave the ideas, worries, and responsibilities of the real world behind. Choose something light that holds your interest but won't put your brain into problem-solving mode. Avoid stressful, violent, or gripping novels.

★ **SLEEP AFFIRMATIONS**: It is easier to sleep when you don't believe in all the negative thoughts you think. Positive affirmations are potent phrases of intent that prompt more helpful thought patterns and perceptions. Choose those meant for relaxation, inner peace, and sleep.

★ **POETRY**: Settle down with a book of healing poems to help you see life through new eyes. Choose something you love to read, something that comforts your heart and opens your mind, even if it's a poem you already know.

★ **SPIRITUAL TEXT**: A collection of poetry, scripture, or mythology—go where your heart is. Touching base with ancient wisdom tunes out modern day stresses and feeds your faith in the unknown.

★ **SACRED MANTRAS**: Meditating on the specific vibrational frequency of a word or set of words is believed to transform consciousness, especially when falling asleep. Consult any spiritual system for a mantra that resonates with you and read it nightly to encourage a healing shift in energy and to transition from one state of consciousness to another.

★ **TAROT, ORACLE, AND HOROSCOPE READINGS**: Card readings are used to explore your innermost self and divine wisdom and guidance. Though each style is different, all three activities can bring a sense of calm and support you through the process of healing, growth, or change. Reading cards is also a time to disconnect from the day and reconnect with yourself.

Build a personal library in a peaceful corner of your home to turn reading time into a ritual you love coming home to.

13. MEDITATIVE COLORING

Coloring is worth exploring long after childhood as a method of replacing stressful thoughts and images with restful ones. Combining elements of art therapy and meditation, the act of focusing on aesthetically-pleasing patterns can reduce tension, induce relaxation, improve vision and attention span, restore feelings of well-being, and prepare you for a deep sleep. This lighthearted activity tunes out chatter and prompts positive neurological responses that elicit a meditation-like state. Whimsical and intricate designs evoke your inner child and provide the freedom to be creative without any real consequence. Even if you don't finish a coloring page before bedtime, the brain enjoys the comfort and predictability of staying inside the lines.

Enjoying the process of choosing and matching colors to shapes is far from elementary: it can be an enchanting and cathartic experience. Difficulties evaporate from your awareness. You give your being an essential respite from external stimuli (news, social highlight reels). Rather than consuming, you are creating—and the gratification of making something beautiful floods you with joy.

Whether you fancy glitter gel pens or good old-fashioned colored pencils, 15 minutes of coloring before bed can contribute to the kind of restoration you've been craving. Explore the charming ritual of coloring your way to sleep:

★ Consciously choose colors that feel calming and pleasant to you. Dark, pastel, and cool colors tend to communicate softer energy than bright colors.

★ Choose themes and designs that encourage a peaceful state of mind. The symmetrical structure of geometric patterns and circular mandalas are especially soothing. To encourage sleepy mental imagery, consider templates of flickering candles, warm beverages, cozy blankets, enchanting nature scenes, starry skies, or positive affirmations.

★ Create a relaxed environment: play soft or whimsical music; light a candle; turn off devices or leave them in another room; diffuse comforting essential oil blends.

★ Make it a shared experience. Color alongside your loved ones, each with your own template or with everyone contributing to one creation.

★ Set an intention before you begin coloring for how you want this process to feel. Surrender the outcome and agree to devote yourself completely to this one experience.

★ As you color, engage your senses. Notice the colors that resonate with you, imagining that each color signifies something positive: peace, love, intuition, etc. Connect to the physical feeling of holding the utensil in your hand as you pick it up and press it into the page. Look and listen for the subtleties.

Revel in the total immersion of coloring. Feel the flow of creating not just a picture but an experience that is always unique. Connecting to your creative inner essence and the pulse of the present moment is a precious gift and a promise of peace.

CHAPTER 8

DREAMY VISUALIZATIONS

The visualization techniques in this chapter involve creating a detailed mental image of a pleasing and peaceful environment, which then becomes a learned cue for the mind and body to prepare for restful sleep. They are essentially suggestions for the mind to explore a more relaxing reality. Spending just a few minutes in reverie can help you detach from ordinary thoughts—reducing stress, soothing anxiety and depression, and enhancing feelings of well-being—and thereby remove some of the common obstacles to getting a peaceful night's rest.

Visualization is an extremely portable tool for achieving better sleep—a healthy outlet for the imagination and an alternative to worrying. With repetition, your capacity for *helpful* creative exploration will expand. Use the following guidelines to support that journey:

★ Create a relaxing external environment where you can practice in peace. Wear loose clothing. Limit distractions. Match scents and sounds to imagery. Consciously relax your body before and during the practice (i.e., it's okay to make adjustments in the middle of a visualization).

★ If stressful thoughts appear, simply imagine what it would look and feel like if those thoughts went away. Ponder how your muscles, heart, belly, and head would feel. This in itself is a *feeling* visualization.

★ You can imagine anything, provided that it contributes to the feeling of relaxation.

★ Immerse yourself in the experience. Consult at least three of your senses to notice as many details as you can: colors, temperature, subtle sounds, scents, tastes, shapes, textures. With practice, you will be able to keep adding details. *Be* in this place.

★ If you find a safe place for sleeping in your mind's eye, you can imagine yourself staying there through the night (rather than coming out of the visualization before bedtime).

★ Practice consistently and indefinitely. Release expectations of immediate relief in the beginning. It may take weeks or months to reprogram old patterns and transport yourself swiftly into a new state of mind, but this will happen with patience and devotion.

Enjoy using your mind in a new way: to retreat into a dreamy place.

1. VISITING YOUR HAPPY PLACE

Use this relaxation script to mentally transport yourself to a pleasant setting—where peace is the most natural thing in the world. Choose anything that pleases you: a private beach, castle in the mountains, field of wildflowers, enchanted forest, spa, temple, cave of crystals, favorite room, and so on. Spending a long moment in your "happy place" prompts your brain to release serotonin, which feels good and helps override old panic patterns, carving a more positive pathway. You're not avoiding but learning to more gracefully cope with stress so that it doesn't control your sleep. The practice can do wonders for soothing insomnia and restlessness.

Follow along to create the perfect place in your mind, where you can retreat before bed and evoke calm at any time:

1. Craft the most peaceful external setting possible. Sit tall or lie down comfortably. Support yourself with blankets and pillows.

2. Close your eyes. Spend a few moments focusing on your breathing, gradually relaxing every muscle. Alternatively, practice a calming meditation or a deep breathing exercise before continuing.

3. If you find it difficult to conjure up pleasing imagery right away, focus on the journey there: the climb up to the top of the mountain; paddling across the lake; anything that resonates with you. This journey takes real effort, but you understand its purpose: reaching your destination. Each step puts distance between you and ordinary life.

4. Imagine coming across a protective archway made of light. It keeps the outside world at bay and provides entrance to

deep restfulness. Come through the archway, leaving the excitement of the journey behind.

5. As you come through, imagine yourself in the most beautiful, serene location, where everything is as you would ideally have it be: your happy place.

6. Immerse yourself in the sensory elements of this place. For instance, vividly imagine the warmth of the sun on your skin and the sound of waves rolling in to the shore. Feel the rich earth beneath your feet and the gentle breeze moving through your hair. Smell the incense in the temple. Hear the birdsong. Run your fingertips along the crystals.

7. Remain in this healing space for as long as you like, whether just a few minutes or 30 minutes.

8. If thoughts from the day appear, gently return your focus to the visualization. You can imagine the thought being carried away in a bubble or by a bird.

9. Before leaving, assure yourself that you can return to this place whenever you wish. You know the way here and it will quietly await your return. Take a mental snapshot of your scene, capturing an image for easy recall after opening your eyes.

10. Gently bring your focus back to your breathing. Open your eyes when ready.

2. MANIFESTING YOUR IDEAL LIFE

According to the universal Law of Attraction, the essence of what you focus on and feel is attracted to you. Thus, when you form clear mental images of what you desire and practice feeling the fruition of those desires, you water the roots of the flower that has yet to bloom. Consider this visualization a tool for *allowing* rather than *achieving* your ideal life. There is a strong emotional element involved that naturally promotes peace in the present moment, clears the clutter from your mind, and improves your outlook. The healing and supportive words, images, and emotions you evoke facilitate positive transformation here and now, making restful sleep a brighter reality.

Use this script to open your heart to receive what you need and to embrace sleep as your most supportive tool in living your dreams:

1. Create a cozy and uplifting external space: burn incense; invite crystals; play music.

2. Affirm your readiness and willingness to co-create what you desire with the universe with something like "I graciously open my heart to receive what feels most loving to me."

3. Choose one or two words that capture what your ideal life would feel like: bliss, freedom, harmony, joy, love, peace, wellness, wholeness, wonder, and so on.

4. Close your eyes. Sit comfortably with your spine tall. Put one hand on your heart and the other on your belly. Take a few deep breaths.

5. Reflect on any images and circumstances that emerge from what these words mean to you. Choose what feels really good. Be specific: the universe responds well to clarity and direction.

6. Picture all the atoms in the universe that resonate with your feelings and visions being magnetically drawn to you. The essence of what you desire most is being delivered. Everything unfolds perfectly.

7. Imagine that you are now living your ideal life. Focus on what you see, what you are doing, and how much you love your life. See yourself happy, whole, and healthy. Immerse yourself in the sensations and the feelings. Breathe in the energy of this space.

8. Focus on what is fulfilling and inspiring about having received everything you want and need to live your dreams.

9. Affirm: "This is my life. This is my truth."

10. Take a few deep breaths. Open your eyes when ready.

11. Carry this feeling and pleasing imagery into bed. To empower what you enjoyed most, write it down in your journal. Allow your dreams to navigate the details of the journey, mining answers and insight so you don't have to. Affirm in writing, out loud, or silently: "I allow what I need to come to me through sleep."

12. Fall asleep with an open heart, knowing you will receive what you need—because you already have.

3. CHOOSING YOUR DREAMS

Visualizations help you break unconscious behavior and thought patterns both in your waking and dreaming states. Like daydreaming at night, this method brings in some elements of lucid dreaming techniques to help you welcome positive experiences into your dreams tonight. Whether or not you want to consciously experience your dreams, this technique can smooth the transition from awake to dreaming. It can be performed simply for its relaxing effects on the mind and body.

Keep a dream journal by your bedside and "choose your dreams" immediately before going to bed or upon waking in the middle of the night. If you do wake up at night, use the disturbance as an opportunity to imagine your way back into a sleeping state of consciousness. In this way, insomnia becomes an invitation to lucid dreaming.

Building your desired dreamscape involves imagination and patience. With practice, you will discover what supports the process and works best for you. The following method will help you begin your journey inward:

1. In your dream journal, plan the main event of tonight's dream. This doesn't need to be a lengthy description and can be bulleted with keywords. Be as detailed as possible and write in the present tense as if the dream is happening right now. Describe your location, scents, sounds, textures, what you are doing and who you are with. You can draw pictures.

2. When finished, snuggle into bed and assume a comfortable position. Close your eyes. Take deep breaths and consciously relax every muscle, one at a time.

3. Bring into your mind's eye the scene you would like to begin your dream with. Again imagine as many small details as possible: Are you running, walking, swimming, sitting, flying? Where are you and what do you see around you? Can you taste something? Are there any noticeable smells? Notice what textures and surfaces you feel. Listen to the subtle sounds in your environment.

4. Notice especially how it feels to be here. Relax into the feeling state of your dreamscape. You can think something like "It feels so good to be here" as you feel your way through every detail.

5. As you feel your body at the threshold of sleep, mentally repeat the phrase "I know I am dreaming" or "This is a dream." Like a mantra, let this one thought scroll through your mind as you continue exploring your dream state.

TIP

You may consider using auditory brainwave entrainment (such as binaural beats therapy, which features pulsing sounds) to support your visualization and induce a dreamlike state of consciousness. Since this method produces different experiences, research or seek medical advice before trying. Playing nature sounds or mystical music can also support specific imagery.

Chapter 8

4. PROGRESSIVE MUSCLE VISUALAXATION

Progressive muscle relaxation involves consciously tensing and relaxing one muscle at a time until the whole body is relaxed. It is a tried-and-true technique for preventing and easing mild to moderate anxiety and depression and encouraging healthier sleep cycles. Bowing to the traditional relaxation technique, this practice brings in a strong element of imagery for a deeply healing experience. The goal is to associate the sensations of physical calm with the visual created in the mind's eye. As you gain practice, sessions involving imagery alone will prompt the body to relax.

For tonight, enjoy the sweeter slumber that follows this "visualaxation":

1. Enter a comfortable position, lying down or sitting. Close your eyes. Tune in to your breathing, letting it naturally slow and lengthen.

2. Inhale through your nose for 3–4 seconds as you squeeze your toes. Visualize tension bottling up in this area, as if your breath is rallying every bit of unease from the surrounding muscles, joints, tendons, and ligaments. If you feel uncomfortable, hold for a lesser count.

3. Exhale slowly and audibly as you release. Imagine sending this concentrated tension through your skin and away to be absorbed into the ether. Sigh it out into the night. Everything you don't need is lifted from this area.

4. On your resting inhale (or two), imagine golden light (or another calming color, such as amethyst or lavender) rushing in to fill this newly created space. It dissolves any remaining discomfort and heaviness.

5. On your resting exhale (or two), let this light soak into your muscles and bathe every nearby cell.

6. Repeat this process as you gradually make your way up to your face, stopping to tighten and relax each muscle—calves, shins, knees, thighs, buttocks, abdomen, back, chest, shoulders, fingers, hands, arms, jaw, nose, eyes, forehead. Inhale to gather tension. Sigh to release. Inhale light energy. Exhale and bathe in essential healing.

7. Once complete, return to natural breathing. Imagine your breath flowing in and out through the surface of your entire body. This turns into an easy feeling visualization as old tension leaves in exchange for nurturing energy. Maintain slow, deep, effortless breathing. Notice how your body lightens.

8. When you are ready, gradually shift your attention to the sensations around you. Open your eyes. Give yourself 1–2 minutes before getting up.

With time, just visualizing this tension and release process will be enough to bring your body into a calm state and remind your brain that it is safe to let go and relax.

5. EMOTIONAL LANDSCAPE

Changing the way you see your internal landscape is a powerful way to alter it. This visualization summons your imagination to help you transcend and reinterpret those distressing stories that want to keep you up at night. By gaining an aerial perspective of your emotional landscape, you gain the freedom to discover some relief there. You are essentially rewiring your subconscious mind to observe emotions without giving them the power to set the course for your night. Course-correcting is an invaluable tool for peace.

Read through this sequence before bed to rise above any disquieting emotions and set the stage for a night of real rest:

1. Sit in a comfortable seat and use relaxed breathing.

2. Select an uncomfortable emotion you would like to shift: uncertainty, failure, shame, regret, bitterness, self-doubt, unworthiness, and so on.

3. Imagine yourself sitting, barefoot and relaxed, on the top of a quiet hill or mountainside. Feel the earth beneath you.

4. Invite the discomfort to come forth and present itself to you as a landscape. With as much curiosity as possible, notice what you see from your neutral and elevated state: a dark forest, violent volcano, vast ocean, dry desert, abandoned building, or anything else. Let your intuition guide you—nothing is wrong.

5. Observe the details of the landscape. Is it indoors or outdoors, sparse or full of images? Seek without forcing. You may sense something instead of seeing it. In your mind,

describe what grabs your attention: sights, sounds, shapes, colors, impressions. Everything (even blank space) is meaningful.

6. Notice that you are not the landscape. Recognize that the place presenting itself to you is an internal state of being that you have recently inhabited and are now observing. Feel the relief of detachment.

7. Walk down and explore the landscape—although you are standing in it, you are not the landscape itself. Discover details with interest: terrain, climate, colors, animals, vegetation, and so on.

8. To heighten your exploration, call in a friendly winged creature who is big enough for you to climb on. It agrees to safely bring you up into the sky. Alternatively, enter a hot air balloon or sit on your own personal cloud.

9. Soar up into the clear sky. You now see the landscape of your emotions from a distance. Notice every edge and design. See how different and small everything looks from up here.

10. When you are ready, ask to be safely brought back to the hill or mountain. As your guide leaves you, flying (or floating) smoothly away into the setting sun, close your eyes and sink into the earth. Your awareness is vast now.

11. Bring your focus back to your steady breathing and the present moment. Open your eyes when you are ready.

6. BODY OF WATER

In this visualization, you bring the soothing seascape to your internal landscape. Since your body is made up mostly of water, focusing on the ocean connects you with your own fluid nature and gives way to the deep inner knowing that you are supported in the infinite ocean of consciousness. You are reminded that you are understood, and you are safe here, and you are held while you sleep. You can relax.

Follow these steps to access the stillness beneath the fluctuating mind—it is always here for you:

1. Lie down on the floor or in your bed (see *savasana*, Chapter 5). Use bolsters, blankets, and pillows for comfort. Relax your jaw and part your lips. Soften your tongue and neck. Close your eyes.

2. Take a moment to acknowledge the rivers and brooks that make up your body. Visualize your heart being the ocean where all paths unite.

3. Notice any disturbances coming up from beneath the surface of your heart's ocean. Use the power of your mind to visually calm your ocean until all you see is a smooth surface.

4. As you become still inside, look around and notice that you're floating in a turquoise body of water—a small cove nestled close to shore, enclosed by a natural rock barrier. The water is calm and warm, and light dances across its surface.

5. You can see the ocean floor beneath you, so you gaze down and take in the most beautiful colors of coral—yellow, orange, purple, red, green. Little fish swim leisurely through the seaweed that's swaying ever so gently.

6. A welcome breeze passes by. You face the sky and bask in this pool that seems to have been reserved just for you. Your body is supported so easily as the salt water removes any heaviness from you.

7. A sense of wonder washes over you. Somehow, but surely, you are one with the water, with the slowly setting sun, with the breeze and the coral below. You are in the infinite flow. You feel at home, bathing in this universal pool of oneness.

8. Quietly return inward, gazing at your heart's ocean. Appreciate its vast splendor. Offer gratitude—thanking the sun, the warm water, and any other elements of your visualization that gave you a moment of pure bliss.

9. Come back home to this moment. Feel yourself held by Mother Earth. Feel the connection you share with everything. Wiggle your toes and fingers, and open your eyes when you're ready.

Feel free to explore variations of this visualization. Each time, consider how amazing it is that you are a living, breathing body of water. Keep a spirit of awe alive inside and sleep will come.

7. LUSH FOREST BATHING

Basking in the lush energy of the earth is enough to refresh your mind, body, and soul. In Japan, the ancient practice of forest bathing involves immersing every sense in the forest atmosphere for an experience of complete nourishment. When you can't venture outdoors, retreat to this creative visualization for some of the same benefits: reduced stress, clarity of mind, and overall rejuvenation. Practice whenever you want to tap into a more fluid (easier, lighter) state of mind—the kind that sleep loves to reward.

Follow these steps to summon the generous energy of Mother Earth right where you are. Open up your heart space, attune your senses, and receive her essential nutrients:

1. Sit in an easy cross-legged position or in a chair with spine straight and palms on your thighs. Close your eyes. Breathe three or more gentle, full breaths in and out of your nose. Bring your consciousness inward and come fully into this moment.

2. Imagine that you are entering a lush forest canopy. Look for a place to rest, completely relaxed and receptive to the vital life energy flowing here.

3. Notice all the vivid colors: rich hues of emerald, hints of lime, golden sunlight playing through the leaves, sparkling waterfalls and streams, bright blossoms pushing through the earth, red and purple berries.

4. Notice what sounds you hear: babbling brooks and streams, wind streaming through the trees, branches dancing, birds singing.

5. Notice what you feel: the warm, sweet air that clears your mind, the light breeze in your hair, the dewy moisture that your skin drinks in, the ground feeding your soul. Let everything be easy and effortless as you breathe it in.

6. Root deeply into every sensation all at once now. Feel the earth's wisdom pulsing through you—restoring you, balancing you, relaxing you. Your sensory body revels in the warmth, the sounds, the colors, the sweet scents.

7. Imagine this earthy energy pouring through the crown of your head and bathing your entire spine with healing nectar. You do nothing but absorb this vitality.

8. Bring your attention to your third eye chakra (center of the eyebrows) and take three or more effortless, full breaths before you return to gentle movement and open your eyes. Know that this lavish healing space is always here to support you anytime you call upon it.

TIPS FOR BLISS

To support total immersion in this sleep-welcoming ritual, bring in living plants or pure essential oils of trees, flowers, or fruits: frankincense, sandalwood, fir, cedarwood, spruce, cypress, juniper berry, bergamot, lavender, orange. Play "pink noise" or soothing forest sounds. Sit on an earthing mat.

8. FALLING LEAVES

Finding freedom from your thoughts is possible when you conjure up the deep inner knowing that your thoughts are not *you*. In this practice, you use the mental image of falling leaves to represent the thoughts that come and go. As you realize that neither your identity nor destiny rests with any one thought, you become less burdened by the thoughts that happen to occur and sleep will naturally become much, much easier.

This visualization can be practiced sitting, standing, or lying down with eyes closed. Whenever you notice that your mind is cluttered and not conducive to sleep, use the following steps to guide you to a free and peaceful present moment:

1. With a deep breath, think or speak to yourself: "Stop." Be firm yet compassionate. This is a surprisingly powerful way to interrupt your thoughts. Repeat if needed.

2. With another deep breath, think or speak: "Allow." This cues you to be the witness of your thoughts as they come and go.

3. Close your eyes and visualize yourself sitting, standing, or lying down on a lush bed of grass—perhaps on a blanket or bench. In front of you is a river with trees on either side. Feel yourself here, watching the leaves float by on the water's surface, into and out of your line of vision. Adjust this nature scene so that it suits your current season and climate.

4. See your thoughts now sitting atop the leaves—one thought for each leaf, one leaf for each thought. Thoughts can be spelled out in words or portrayed as an image or sensation.

5. Look at your thoughts. Let them be there. Notice that you are not the thoughts themselves: you are the one looking at them.

6. Now visualize a "thought leaf" as it is dropped from a nearby tree. This leaf comes into your line of vision, swirls in the gentle breeze, and lands in the water. Watch from a distance as it's carried out of sight by the slow current.

7. See each leaf with its thought coming and going. Let it come; let it go. Let another come and watch it float away. You are simply witnessing and allowing.

8. Come back to the mantra of "allow" if you find yourself attaching to any particular thought. Keep returning to this nature scene.

9. Continue until you feel peaceful and at ease with your thoughts being "there" and you being "here."

With practice, you may find that you're able to settle into this visualization with open eyes in a matter of seconds. In that case, move through the rest of your night with this loose mental imagery, infusing peace with every step, all the way to bed.

9. STARRY MIND

If you are craving a connection to everything, look at the night sky. Stargazing is the perfect opportunity to contemplate the ingredients you share with the glistening lights above: you are gazing at the same source of the weightier atoms in your body. There are fragments of stars within you. The reverie this visualization elicits unites you with wonder and leaves you with dreamy imagery and the affirmation that you are worthy of breathing and sleeping in peace. You are an inherent part of the slow dance of life. The solace this perception brings is the stuff of dreams.

1. Connect with the night sky. Go outside, preferably, or look out a window and stargaze for at least 30 seconds and as long as you like. Let this be a quiet, intimate moment. The sky doesn't need to be bright with starlight and a full moon for your eyes to be graced with the magnificence of the cosmos.

2. Inside, create a contemplative space: play celestial music; invite essential oils of patchouli, lavender, frankincense, or cedarwood; cozy up with blankets and pillows as if you were camping outside.

3. Lie down in comfort. Close your eyes when you're settled in. Bring slow, deep breaths into and out of your nose, finding a smooth and easy rhythm.

4. Bring to mind tonight's night sky. See the moon and speckled stars spanning the horizon of your mind, reflected in the pool of your awestruck heart. Your imagery may be more

magical than what you saw outside tonight—enjoy the most spectacular scenic view.

5. Imagine you are lying on the earth, connected above and below to the infinite beauty and marvel of the universe. You are held. You are sustained. You are safe to explore the luminous details of the cosmic ocean in peace.

6. Feel your heart filling with fascination as you pick out the details of your sky: every star, some near and some far; constellations; shooting stars; the phase of the moon; the passing clouds; nightfall unfolding against an indigo backdrop.

7. If a distracting thought appears, picture it swirling like stardust upward into the sky, where it is remade into a shining new star.

8. You might notice fireflies drifting through the air around you or crickets chirping. Welcome any friendly sounds from your cozy spot on the earth.

9. Continue stargazing and soaking up the wondrous healing energy of the natural nightlights all around you. Ponder your shared ingredients with the stars and your essential connection to everything you see, feel, and hear. Stay here for as long as you wish.

10. When you are ready to return indoors, invite small movements into your fingers and toes. Stretch your arms and legs. Open your eyes.

10. THE ALTAR WITHIN

Just as you might create an altar in your home for your devotional practices, the purpose of this visualization is to elevate your internal environment. This ritual takes place in the temple that is your body, home to your heart and soul on earth. You will create mental images of objects that feel soothing and sacred to you—objects you would keep at your home altar—and imagine placing them at the altar of your own heart. This uniquely personal practice encourages feelings of control, confidence, focused attention, spiritual connection, self-compassion, and well-being. Sweeter dreams are only a heartbeat away.

Optional objects for your "inner altar" can include: decorative cloth, crystals, incense, candles, anointing oil, Himalayan salt lamps, mala beads, statues, pictures, poetry, scripture, flowers, other natural elements.

1. Craft a pleasant external environment that is comfortable, free from distraction, and filled with any of your actual altar objects.

2. Find a comfortable, supported position, sitting with a straight spine or lying down. Close your eyes. Consciously relax every muscle in your face and body.

3. Rest your right hand on your heart. Let your left hand rest on the ground (lying down) or on your lap (sitting), palm facing the sky with index finger and thumb gently touching. Alternatively, rest both hands on your heart, right hand underneath left.

4. Take several full belly breaths. Exhale to release ordinary thoughts. Inhale to receive sacred energy. Exhale everyday life. Inhale divine support.

5. Imagine that your body is a temple—indoor or outdoor—filled with everything that enchants and delights the spirit. You might envision rubies and other gemstones laid upon every table, fresh flowers growing from the rich earth, walls lined with beautiful paintings, stained glass windows, or frankincense swirling in the air.

6. Once you have spent ample time painting a mental picture of your temple, silently repeat the mantra "I am the temple."

7. Bring your awareness to your heart: the altar. Notice its size and shape, made from any material that inspires you. Step closer and feel its texture, inspect its uniqueness, praise its beauty, contemplate every curvature. Honor this most sacred place of devotion and divination.

8. Silently repeat the mantra "I am the altar."

9. In your mind, begin bringing up one object at a time to place on or around your altar. Adorn this space with care. Understand this as a powerful offering of love, appreciation, and respect.

10. When you are finished with this ritualistic act, silently repeat the mantra "I am the love."

11. Silently repeat the whole mantra: "I am the temple. I am the altar. I am the love."

12. When ready, bring gentle movement into your body. Breathe deeply. Open your eyes.

Enjoy the beauty sleep that comes when you honor yourself.

11. HEALING ENERGY BLANKET

It is only through your unconditional loving presence that deep healing can occur. This visualization helps you heal wounds and clear negativity without letting the pain consume you. Your imagined "blanket of warm light" provides a very real sense of protection so that you can transform any thought, emotion, or physical hurt that has been causing you unrest. Practice this whole-being treatment to remove residual energy from the day and to protect your energy tonight so that you can instead focus on how good sleep feels. You will set a healthy boundary so that anxiety can melt away and so that peace cannot be taken away.

If something needs resolution, it first needs loving attention and the following steps offer a creative and safe way to do that:

1. Pick a pain point to transform or soften: a physical ailment, a nagging thought, things you can't control, sharp emotions, or the negativity of another person.

2. Breathe deeply into this pain with eyes closed. You don't need to fix or change anything yourself. Simply breathe and ask for assistance.

3. Imagine a blanket made of warm golden light coming to your aid and surrounding this pain point. It creates a protective force field around this thought, feeling, injury, or other person.

4. This blanket is not heavy but light. Imagine it gently extracting the heaviness inside and sending it out to be absorbed by the darkness. Inside its embrace, everything softens.

5. Hold this visual for several breaths or minutes.

6. Envision the light coming to hug your entire body now, forming a cocoon of warm golden awareness around you. Your aura (the field of luminous energy that surrounds you) and every cell are bathed and cleansed. Only the healing qualities of love can enter. You breathe in and out only positive energy.

7. Hold this visual for several breaths. Sink deeper into the experience. Feel this complete and pleasant protection, this liberation and lightness. Feel yourself calm and restored. You may feel as though your body is tingling—mingling with the healing energy of the universe.

8. In your mind's eye, see each exhalation now expanding your bubble of protection until your entire home is blanketed in love. The light of all the stars in the sky shines through to lift away every bit of debris. Stay here for several breaths.

9. When ready, open your eyes. Hold this visual if you like. Know that this healing energy continues to mingle with yours, even while you sleep.

Whenever something painful shows up for you, show up for it with a healing blanket of energy. You can practice this visualization with eyes open once you're familiar with the steps: surround the hurt; surround yourself; surround your home.

12. BLURRED EDGES

Moving through life on "autopilot" leaves much to be desired—connection with your inner voice, with others' hearts, and with the natural energies of the earth. Here is a mindfulness practice to turn down the volume of hurried and anxious thoughts so you can access a fuller state of peace and joy. By becoming fully engaged with your experience of the present moment, you break the chain of mindless action and make a connection with the still place from which sleep flows with ease.

This open-eye visualization brings the power of mindfulness into full effect, right here and right now, igniting the sensation that you are one with everything—from the moonlit sky to your bed. It can be performed alongside many other rituals. Whether you're sweeping the floor, taking a walk, sipping tea, or brushing your teeth, apply the following steps to turn whatever you're experiencing into something reverent:

1. Exhale fully, emptying yourself of air. Inhale deeply, letting your belly expand and fill you with the air around you.

2. Look at one prominent object nearby. This could be the dish you are washing, the food on your plate, the cup you are drinking from, the table you are sitting at, a picture on the wall, a tree or rock—any *thing*.

3. Observe the object with your full focus. See it as though you have never seen it before. Study its features, materials, colors, imperfections: every quality and detail your five senses note.

4. Imagine the edges of this object beginning to soften and fade into the air around them. Hard lines blur and maybe start to shimmer as you imagine tiny particles breaking off from the main body of the object, floating away like stardust into the ether.

5. Stick with this one object. If you can maintain the visual, continue to see every object in this way, one by one, until all the edges of your environment become blurred, dancing, as if they are mingling with the air around them.

6. Bring your attention to your own body and see your edges softening into the world around you. Your spatial awareness becomes expansive. Your blurred edges start to mingle with those of the objects around you.

7. Notice how you and each object share this space, everything "breathing" the same air. Contemplate the depth and breadth of that connection.

8. Hold this visual loosely, if you wish, as you partake in your other evening rituals.

Sensing your intricate connection to everything, surrender to sleep, supported and wholly at ease.

CHAPTER 9

REFLECTING AND RELEASING FOR PEACE

Your brain has a natural tendency to want to remember things. This is why forcing yourself to forget about grievances and worries usually means you end up taking your problems to bed with you. Even today's joys and tomorrow's priorities can keep your brain working overtime making sure nothing is lost. Consider this chapter peace training. These rituals serve as healthy ways to digest thoughts and feelings and disentangle yourself from rumination and expectation. Knowing that you have mentally, emotionally, and spiritually dealt with something frees up precious headspace so you can get more grounded in *this* moment. Leaning in and loosening the grip of every "should" and "should have" means you get to play with another perspective, here and now, and that is where the real transformation happens.

Here are a few thoughts to consider as you document and digest the distressing thoughts and feelings (since those are the ones that can be more difficult to accept and release):

★ Instead of destroying the discomfort, dissolve it in your focused awareness. The less you resist something, the less it controls you and begs you to stay awake contemplating it. You may discover that even heartbreak, frustration, and fear can have valuable messages wrapped up inside of them.

★ Take on the role of "passive observer." Feel the feeling while noticing that it is not your identity. Let it be "there" and let yourself be "here" until you feel a little more wiggle room between it and you.

★ Say goodnight to the experience. Whether you write it down, say it out loud, drop it into a box, burn it, forgive it, or visualize it being dissolved, there is something cathartic about watching what once had such a strong emotional grip on you fade away into the night.

When there's nothing left to forget or remember, all that's left for you to do is relax.

1. EVENING PAGES

Everything you keep to yourself takes up cognitive resources. This is why expressive writing is so good for your mental health and your sleep—it keeps your brain from feeling like it has to juggle (and replay) everything. Whether you are struggling with a decision, craving self-acceptance, grieving, or stuck on a nagging thought, Evening Pages is a ritual that meets you where you are. It is a safe outlet for processing emotions, enhancing self-awareness, and trying on a fresh perspective. Like a data dump, the practice takes an "anything goes" approach: write until you feel the release.

Through these inward explorations, you practice courage and get better at disputing false evidence appearing real—F.E.A.R. You might even stumble upon some hidden gems in the process, like forgotten strength or a new opportunity. The goal isn't to write well but to get what's inside out. Whatever shows up on the page, notice how there is that much more space inside your head and heart.

Experiment with the following suggestions to make the most out of this humble tool for peaceful sleep:

★ Write about goals, troubles, joys, worries, even sleep—journaling signals to the brain that what you're writing about is important, so it seeks out supportive resources and relevant opportunities to meet your needs. It seems counterintuitive, but even as you transcribe your fears, you are less likely to worry because it's being taken care of.

★ Greet discomfort, boredom, confusion, and fear of the blank page with compassionate awareness, curiosity, messy imperfection, patience, and a willingness to write whatever comes up. It might help to write quickly (stream of consciousness style) to prevent over-analyzing and self-micromanagement.

★ Be brutally, beautifully honest. Flow without a filter. Paper is forgiving.

★ No fancy notebook is needed, but make sure it's something you love to write in—same goes for what you write with.

★ It is okay if it looks like furious scribbling, as long as it feels like freedom—better the fury on paper where you can look at it from a distance than caged inside your head and heart.

★ Treat every fear or painful occurrence with questions, like "What do you want to show me? How can I see this differently? How can you help me?"

★ Set up a safe and supportive environment: turn on a Himalayan salt lamp, play relaxing music, light a candle, slip under a blanket, or sip from your favorite mug.

It is a comfort to fall asleep knowing all of your thoughts and feelings have been tucked away, safely held for you, in between the pages of your journal. You just gave yourself permission to enjoy the simplicity of the present moment.

2. GRATITUDE JOURNALING

For a grateful heart and a calm mind, pause. A steady gratitude journaling practice helps you to tap into the subtle gifts that often go unnoticed in a busy world. By slowing down at night, you recapture the beauty and small victories of the day. This lends a calmer energy that's conducive to sleep, as you're eased into a state of joy, connectedness, fulfillment, and peace.

Positive psychology research shows gratitude to be directly correlated with greater happiness and overall well-being. It can support your ability to relish positive experiences, build strong relationships, deal with adversity, and find closure. Since positive thinking fuels its own forward motion, expressing gratitude helps reprogram thoughts to break negative cycles— the ones that keep you awake at night. Writing down new thoughts deepens their emotional impact and thus consciously giving thanks on paper retrains your brain and changes you. You'll not just seek out things to be grateful for tonight, either; you'll grow more apt to seek them out during the day.

Your thanks don't need to be profound or complex to set a positive cycle in motion, just sincere and felt. No blessing is too small.

Topics you can write about tonight include:

* Gifts/blessings received, material or otherwise
* How you were able to contribute or help someone
* Things that did or did not happen
* Meaningful lessons learned and challenges overcome
* Unexpected positive events, humor, beauty, or grace
* What is working well in your life

Here are some helpful tips on keeping a gratitude journal for nightly soothing:

★ For consistency and fluidity, dedicate a separate journal or section in your current journal to gratitude.

★ Write with awareness and intention. It's not about counting your blessings like sheep but thoughtfully engaging with them as you transcribe them. Immerse yourself. Be one with the moment and the message.

★ Write three to five detailed entries. One sentence each will suffice, though you can write lengthier passages. Be as detailed as possible about *why* you are grateful.

★ Research varies on the effectiveness of daily versus weekly journaling. Find the frequency that works for you, and keep entries specific to that day/week.

★ Date and number pages. It's inspiring to reflect on past thanks and encouraging to see how far you have come.

★ Doodle. Drawings can help solidify your gratitude (and you don't need to be an artist).

Writing down grateful thoughts opens the door to the true riches in life that were previously hiding in plain sight. Pause to reflect and explore, and you'll be a magnet for sound sleep.

3. FORGIVENESS LETTERS

Forgiveness is the practice of softening your need for a different past. Instead, you place your point of power in the present moment. It is a conscious, ongoing decision to devote more energy to loving your life, here and now, than to feeding the energy of the initial insult. The *willingness* to forgive can exist even when you are not ready to forgive: it is the opening from which a life-enriching practice can grow. Writing a forgiveness letter is a courageous way to close the day and gift yourself the emotional and spiritual freedom that you deserve. The sense of psychological closure lowers the tendency to dwell on hurtful events and makes it easier to invest your precious energy in tonight's peace. Through this practice, you author a night with less anxiety and greater confidence in your ability to receive restful sleep.

Nighttime is the perfect time to take your power back—this does not necessarily mean you need to forgive and forget. What you can do is choose not to allow pain to take up permanent residence in your heart. To help you transform pain into peace, think of this exercise as purely for your own good.

To begin, try writing about an event that you don't feel quite so strongly about. Starting "easy" will naturally lead to the resolution of more difficult cases over time.

1. Recall the incident. Allow yourself a full 90 seconds to feel the emotions (setting a timer might help).

2. Write about what happened and why it still causes you pain. Explain what you wish had happened instead.

3. Describe what could have caused the perpetrator to cause harm. Identify the factors, beliefs, or circumstances that might have influenced or even pressured this person to act in the way that they did.

4. Close your letter with a variation of this statement: "I realize now that what you did was the best you could do through your level of consciousness at that time in your life. For the sake of my own peace, I (am willing to) forgive you. With this act, I consider this incident closed (for tonight)."

You can write this letter to another person or to your past self. You can even imagine writing to their innermost or "higher" self. Remember that truly happy people do not intentionally cause harm and what is not an act of love is a call for love. For more difficult cases, you may need to perform this ritual several times before the grudge releases its grip on you. It may help to practice a heart-opening meditation (see Lovingkindness [Metta] Meditation in Chapter 7) or a Self-Loving Oil Massage (see Chapter 3) first.

4. LETTERS FROM THE SKY

In this comforting writing exercise, you answer your own "prayers" from the point of view of some higher intelligence—from the perspective of the sky. It is essentially like dipping your fingertips in a pool of wisdom and then writing to yourself from that place. The process gets you out of your own head and reminds you that you are not blocked from what you need: guidance, peace, patience, sleep. Feeling as though you are beautifully entangled with everything is a salve and a sedative for the mind, body, and soul.

1. Create a comfortable atmosphere where you can sit and feel supported and safe. Bring in several blankets or a weighted blanket, turn on a Himalayan salt lamp, diffuse a soothing essential oil blend, or anything else that helps.

2. In a journal that is separate from your other writing exercises, open to a blank page.

3. Before you write anything, close your eyes and summon assistance from above. You can ask the moon and stars, a loved one who has passed, the universe, or any higher power of your own understanding to communicate with you. Ask for a compassionate observation from the sky related to any specific or general discomfort or struggle that you need help with.

4. Let yourself be open to the process of asking and listening for answers. Trust in the intelligence that wants to come through to greet you on this page. Be curious and confident in your connection. Listen in a meditative state for as long as you need to.

5. At the top of the page, write an introduction: "Dear soul, this is what I/we would most like you to know tonight…" or "Dear guide, I welcome you to write through me now."

6. When you are ready, begin writing a letter to yourself, in the second person, from the point of view of the sky. Imagine yourself rising way up above all of your concerns tonight. What comfort or hope might that greater perspective grant you? Write from that place.

7. Write slowly or quickly, capturing words, feelings, or visions. Your handwriting might change. You might feel a presence of energy or change in temperature move through you.

8. Close your eyes at any time to better sense the messages.

9. When you feel that you are finished, close your eyes and thank your guide in the sky for helping you tonight. Close your journal with a sigh of relief. Relax into a state of surrender.

It can help to ground yourself in your body after this exercise: stretch; sip tea (see Chapter 4); take a bath (see Chapter 3). Falling asleep is a near-magical experience when you trust that all is well—as above, so below.

5. MINDING A PEACE JAR

When you pay attention to something, you feed that experience. Creating a peace jar is an accessible way to collect the quiet and beautiful moments of your day—the experiences that feel good to feed—making it that much easier to unlock the gates to a peaceful slumber tonight. The practice bolsters positive mental habits by bringing your attention to those smaller moments that tend to slip by unnoticed. By engaging in this ritual, you champion the very emotions, sensations, and thoughts that are going to help you settle into a state of contentment. You turn otherwise forgotten or underestimated moments into serene memories. Something else you'll come to notice is that serenity is about one step away from sound sleep.

You will need:

- ★ A vessel of any shape and material (feel free to decorate, or not)
- ★ A pen, pencil, or marker that you love to use
- ★ Plain, pretty, new, or scrap paper
- ★ A safe and accessible location, such as your nightstand or altar

Each night, mindfully jot down a simple moment worth noticing/cherishing on a piece of paper and drop it into the jar. Pull from the jar on those nights when you could use a lift. Whether you turn this ritual into the act of replenishing or pulling from your jar, you are reinforcing an experience of peace—there is no one "right way," only the way that feeds your soul tonight.

It's those small, everyday marvels that, when you spend some time reconnecting with them, plant peace in your soul. Here are just a few examples of what you might recover or discover in your peace jar:

★ Tiny moments of awe, joy, connection, and gratitude that you want to savor

★ Goals accomplished and small victories

★ Loving "notes to self" (themes of forgiveness and acceptance may come up)

★ Prompts that stimulate feel-good thoughts and emotions, such as "It is time to dream beautiful things" or "What would Love do?"

★ Ways you have grown, lessons learned, and fears overcome

★ Words of wisdom or encouragement

★ Positive affirmations or quotes

★ Favorite verses of poetry or scripture

Let this be a time of devotion and discovery. Rather than rushing through this like an ordinary routine, transform it into a ritual through your loving attention. Recall the moment as if you were there again, and let the wonder of it wash over you. Let it fill your heart with gladness. This is how you bring peaceful moments of the past into the present, and present-moment peace into tomorrow.

6. LETTING GO WITH A UNIVERSE BOX

A universe box is a powerful way to practice surrendering attachments for the sake of peace. If you're struggling with a particular thought or concern tonight, a universe box can help you let it go: yesterday's grudges and regrets; today's frustrations and failures; tomorrow's confusion and worries; and any experience you're holding that keeps you from feeling good and free. As a nightly ritual, it builds a foundation of present-moment contentment and trust—a recipe for peaceful sleep.

All you need to begin is a vessel of your own liking, paper, a writing utensil, and something you're willing to be helped with. Each night, drop a handwritten note into the vessel, offering thanks for or summoning spiritual assistance. You don't need to adopt a new belief system: you are simply opening yourself up to receive the guidance of a higher power of your own understanding, a universal plan, or the same cosmic intelligence that makes the flowers bloom. The only beliefs you're asked to "give up" are those that are blocking you from inner ease.

When you request a higher power or plan to take care of the things you can't or don't need to control, you trade force for peace. You are offering thanks for the guidance you'll ultimately receive, which makes it easier to receive—answers, opportunities, and a good night's sleep. The willingness to ask is the willingness to receive.

Here are some useful tips for creating and using a universe box for serenity and sound sleep:

★ Identify what's blocking you. Be as specific as you can.

★ Experiment with opening statements such as "Thank you, universe, for helping me…" or "Dear universe, please take away my need to…"

★ Ask or give thanks for something that will benefit not just you, but everyone involved. The best way to get out of your own way is to request universal assistance and the best way to get out of the universe's way is to summon a solution that serves the greatest good.

★ Surrender in faith, not defeat. You're not giving up; you're offering *it* up so that it can be reorganized and reinterpreted for you.

★ As you drop in each note, imagine that your request is already in the process of being answered.

★ Trade your plan for a higher plan. Though you may not see or hear a solution right away, trust that you've been heard and what you need will arrive exactly when your soul is ready to receive it.

The physical act of writing down what's bothering you and offering it up to a grand support system feeds your faith that all really is well—and it's okay to get some rest while you're being taken care of.

7. CUTTING ENERGETIC CORDS

When a relationship is initiated, energetic ties are activated. The ceremonial ritual of "cord cutting" is based on the premise that every interaction, thought, and emotion is stored in this etheric cord connecting two people. Whereas a healthy cord enables a vibrant exchange of energy, an unhealthy cord can leave you feeling drained or controlled—even if the relationship has ended. By removing the weight (and distraction) of unpleasant attachments, you can return to a peaceful state that's more conducive to sleep.

Cutting energetic cords is an act of freedom for both sides, including those you care for. This is not an attack but rather a therapeutic exercise for preserving *your* energy. Positive ties of love and respect remain; only those that cause suffering are released.

1. Sit in an easy pose, shoulders and jaw soft, palms on your thighs, breathing relaxed, eyes closed.

2. Visualize yourself in a safe and healing place, real or imagined.

3. Summon spiritual assistance (angels, guides, the cosmos). Speak or think an invocation, something like "I call upon you for healing guidance and protection. Help me release this recurring negative/needy energy that is not serving me."

4. Invite the person with whom you feel a heavy connection into your mind's eye. See them standing before you. Feel the judgment or discomfort.

5. See a thick, dark cord connecting you. Notice where you see and feel it: navel, heart, throat, third eye, or elsewhere.

6. Express how you feel with authority (out loud or silently). You are not justifying grudges—you are illuminating them. Feel the supportive presence of spirit.

7. Hold a luminous crystal sword in your dominant hand. Hold the cord in your free hand. Prepare to clear the slate and release all pent-up energies. Speak an affirmative statement such as "I cut this cord of unhealthy attachment with you."

8. Raise your sword and bring it down as you effortlessly slice through the cord, watching it fall to the ground. What remains dissolves into the night sky, scattering like stardust.

9. Empowered, request that your guardian return to you any lost positive energy. Watch the area where the cord once was being filled with healing light.

10. See the person standing in their innocence as a pure expression of life. Offer your forgiveness: their freedom from you means that *you* are freed.

11. Inhale fully and sigh with relief. You are no longer entangled in this energetic relationship. Open your eyes when ready.

If there are strong emotional undercurrents, you may need to repeat this exercise whenever you feel the need. You don't need to share this with the other person: this is your personal practice for inner peace. You might feel lighter, balanced, or exhausted. Follow with a cleansing ritual or prepare for deep sleep.

8. FIRE RELEASE CEREMONY

Burning ceremonies have long been used to clear away unwanted energies, attachments, emotions, and patterns and create space for new possibilities. The physical act of burning offers a sense of closure and hope—two things that naturally invite rest. New moons and full moons are excellent times for a potent practice, but you can perform this ritual whenever you strongly desire a positive shift away from burdensome patterns and toward healthier sleep patterns.

For a safe outdoor ceremony, you will need:

* ★ Paper or bay leaves
* ★ A writing utensil
* ★ A match or lighter
* ★ Long tongs
* ★ A burn-friendly space: open fire pit, stone or dirt clearing
* ★ If burning in a clearing, a fire-resistant container to catch ashes: cast iron pot, kitchen cauldron, stone dish, terra-cotta pot, metal or glass bowl
* ★ A way to extinguish the flame if necessary: jug of water, fire extinguisher (use fire precautions)

Perform your fire release ceremony with compassion and care—do not burn in the heat of the moment. If needed, meditate your way into a calm mindset before beginning.

1. Create an outdoor altar with candles, natural elements, and anything that calls to be a part of the experience.

2. Close your eyes. Visualize each inhale drawing down cosmic assistance and each exhale rooting you firmly in the earth's

embrace. Repeat for several breaths until you feel focused and grounded.

3. Write down what you wish to release: habits, beliefs, wounds—one thing for each slip of paper or leaf. Be clear and sincere.

4. Read what you've written. Notice every emotion, memory, thought, or sensation that comes up. Feeling it will empower the release.

5. Hold one piece of paper or leaf with tongs over your container or fire pit and ignite. As you burn each item, affirm what you are releasing with something like "I release you. You are free." Envision the fire dissolving all blockages and old ways.

6. When you have finished burning all items, gaze into the fire and pause to revel in any shift you feel.

7. Extinguish the flame, thanking the fire for performing its alchemy. Watch the smoke carry away old energy and all attachment—good and bad. Allow the universe to provide for you in its own creative way.

8. If there are ashes, bury them in the earth or scatter them in a forest to provide fertile ground from which new opportunities can rise. Make sure they are cool—douse with water first for safety.

For a fireless release ceremony, drop torn pieces of paper or leaves into your cauldron and bury them when finished. If your heart is in the practice, it is perfect. As the last of your expectations disperse, fall asleep trusting that all is well and you are supported.

9. TAPPING FOR PEACE

Self-limiting thoughts and their emotions manifest in the body, showing up as pain, tightness, or unrest. A little release could mean an easier night's sleep. Tapping is a powerful holistic stress-release technique also known as Emotional Freedom Technique (EFT). The process involves using your fingers to stimulate acupressure points while talking through your emotions. Giving a voice to the tape that's playing in your head unveils the source of tension; at the same time, the physical "percussion" tells the brain that you are safe and it's okay to relax. This marriage of psychology and acupressure neutralizes any judgment around your stressful thoughts so that there's space for positive and peaceful change.

Move through the following nine acupressure points while speaking your mind:

1. **KARATE CHOP POINT**: On the side of either hand, underneath the pinky.

2. **EYEBROW**: On the bone where the hair of your eyebrow begins.

3. **SIDE OF THE EYE**: Not the temple, but the bone on the side of your eye.

4. **UNDER THE EYE**: On the bone.

5. **UNDER THE NOSE**: Above your lips.

6. **CHIN**: On the crease between your chin and lower lip.

7. **COLLARBONE**: On each side, under your clavicles. You can use your whole hand to tap.

8. **UNDER THE ARM**: About a hand's width from either armpit.

9. **TOP OF THE HEAD.**

Speaking out loud adds another level of concentration, but you can repeat silently. Use the following guidelines, moving through as many rounds of tapping as you need for relief:

1. Check in with your body. Notice where you feel tension or pain. Rate this tension on a scale of 1 to 10.

2. Take a long, deep inhale and exhale.

3. While tapping on the karate chop point, start with a setup statement, filling in your own blank: "Even though..." followed up by the issue, then "I accept how I feel" or "I love and accept myself." For example: "Even though I feel stressed, I love and accept myself." Repeat three times.

4. Continue tapping on each acupressure point while honestly expressing in detail how you feel and why. For example, tap on the points with phrases like: "I feel all this stress... I don't know how to let go... There is too much to do... but right now, I am safe... I can accept myself... It is okay to relax."

5. When your practice feels complete, notice any change and rate your tension again. You can write down any insights or stories that came up.

With practice, you will be able to think and speak about what's bothering you without having the stressful physical response. That is where the shift happens and new, empowering thoughts have a chance to stick and bring you more confidently in the direction of sleep.

10. NURTURING CONVERSATIONS

Taking time to strengthen your closest relationships will help you rest peacefully knowing you have given and received love today. What better way to end your day than surrounded by love? Basking in the joy of good company may also play an integral role in your happiness. The intimacy of touch or close physical presence cues your body to release the hormone oxytocin, which makes you feel happy and lessens the effects of stress, fear, and pain. It is much easier to fall asleep with joy in your heart.

Focus on the snug, comfortable, down-to-earth, friendly kinds of conversation to get the love flowing. Make it a nightly or weekly tradition to greet each other on a deeply nurturing level. Let this be a chance to swap stories and dreams: What went well today? What are you each grateful for? What acts of kindness did you see or participate in? What are you excited about doing better tomorrow?

Put your phones down and be there for each other—wholeheartedly, curiously. Your "meeting of hearts" is a precious opportunity to cultivate compassion, to recover and discover what you love about each other and about life.

Consult the following suggestions to help you build and maintain a warm and safe atmosphere that's conducive to sleep:

★ Be authentic. To give and receive honest support and to be wholly understood, you must allow yourself to *be yourself.* Set the intention to share thoughts and feelings with openness and sincerity.

★ Demonstrate equality. Let there be a lot of relaxed thoughtfulness where nobody dominates the conversation for long stretches of time.

★ Touch them with your presence. Put your arm around them, touch their hand or shoulder—even if you don't make physical contact, let your awareness communicate that they are heard and seen. Practice emulating the yogic phrase *namaste*, which means "the light in me honors the light in you" or simply, "I see you."

★ If you catch yourself formulating a response while someone else is talking, come back to their words and listen just to listen.

★ Practice patience by consciously accepting each other's imperfections. This could also be called *showing some grace*. Give each other the freedom to be human. Soften your expectations.

★ Offer words of affirmation. Share your gratitude for their presence, what qualities you admire, what they did that you enjoyed, benefited from, or were inspired by today.

In place of engaging with another human being tonight, you can talk to, play with, and cuddle your animal companions. This invites the same loving energy to flow through you, helping decrease tension and lower blood pressure (two magnets for sound sleep).

11. MIRROR GAZING

One of the greatest gifts you can give yourself is your own unwavering attention. Looking into the mirror before bed and offering yourself that grace is a therapeutic path to getting the sleep your whole being is seeking. It might feel awkward and silly at first, and you don't need to be in love with yourself to practice, but a steady practice will have some loving consequences. This is the thing: supportive self-talk is important because you are always listening to and processing the stories you tell yourself. The energy of self-rejection likely isn't serving deep restoration. Purposely being on your own team is like giving yourself permission to receive a good night's sleep.

The purpose of mirror gazing is to purify the way you see yourself—without needing to distort, avoid, or condemn what shows up. This is a precious opportunity to meet unloving ways with a new way: love where it's due. As you trade judgment for acceptance, your mind takes a break from chasing painful stories to a logical conclusion. It takes courage to show up like this. There is no healing practice like it.

Use these tips to practice looking in the mirror and loving yourself to sleep:

★ Imagine you are speaking to a friend who is feeling what you are feeling. What would you say? Perhaps: "I am here for you. What do you need? How can I help?"

★ Greet your soul. In Sanskrit, *namaste* (nah-mah-stay): "I honor your light." In Zulu, *sawubona* (sow-boh-nah): "I see you." In Hawaiian, *ho'oponopono* (ho-o-pono-pono): "I love you. I'm sorry. Please forgive me. Thank you."

★ Speak an affirmation that feels better and is accessible enough to repeat. If "I love and accept you" feels unreachable, try something like "I am learning to see you with compassion" or "You might actually be enough."

★ Ponder the life your body has enabled you to experience. Look at yourself like maybe you are here as you are because you are supposed to be here as you are.

★ Consider how every circumstance is specifically designed to bring to the surface what most needs your love.

★ Refer to yourself in the third person as if your challenges are someone else's challenges. This creates psychological distance from what's bothering you, making space for solutions.

★ Honor your future self. Your new peaceful patterns will serve you tonight and thus tomorrow, tomorrow night, and so on.

As you continue to meet yourself, the mirror becomes a chance for self-exploration and validation instead of condemnation. Consciously repeat an empowering story enough and it weaves itself into your identity.

12. WHISPERING PRAYER

Building a relationship with the Divine (or whatever name resonates with you) is a lullaby for the soul. The weight of perfection and everyday living is lifted and replaced with something that could be called grace. As one of the most widespread and time-honored traditions, nightly prayer is a practical way to facilitate healing and inner strength—spiritual, mental, emotional, and physical—even if you are not religious. If you open your mind and heart, you might find this ritual to be a rich and illuminating companion on your journey "back home" to inner peace and deep sleep.

Similar to meditation, prayer can alleviate symptoms of stress, anxiety, depression, physical pain, insomnia, and chronic illnesses such as heart disease and cancer. It could be the combination of spirituality and concentrated focus that elicits the relaxation response, which bolsters immunity, slows heart rate, lowers blood pressure, steadies the breath, and fosters a tranquil alertness. On top of that, the release of dopamine encourages a sense of radiant well-being and joy. In a nutshell, you are equipped to release worry and distraction when it's time for bed.

Here are some sample universal prayers best whispered to draw you inward to a peaceful state of mind that is receptive to sleep—adjust according to your beliefs as needed:

★ **LOVINGKINDNESS (METTA) PRAYER**: May all beings be peaceful. May all beings be happy. May all beings be safe. May all beings be free.

★ **GRATITUDE**: Thank you for another chance to open my heart and feel differently. Thank you for this breath and the chance to see differently. I am willing to believe in all the blessings that are in store for me.

★ **DIVINE DIRECTION**: I am ready to receive all the guidance and grace of the cosmos. May the light of the stars plant faith in my heart. I am willing to trust in the creative solutions that are meant for me.

★ **PEACE**: May my inner reservoir of peace be plenty. May my body be nourished while I sleep. May I be guided to tranquility inside. May my heart be comforted and freed from every blockage to peace.

★ **HEALING**: Please help me to know forgiveness so that I can be healed. Let love be all that I remember tonight. I surrender to the journey back home to wholeness. I am ready to dissolve all barriers to healing in your light.

Prayer is a highly intuitive and intensely personal practice. Whichever words you choose to whisper before bed, let them be genuine. Allow your prayer to come from your heart to the heart of your Source, your inner wellspring of peace that lives underneath everything.

APPENDIX: RITUAL SEQUENCES

The moon has her phases and so do you. While each phase (or season) carries its own energy, lessons, and obstacles, you do not need to be anyone or anywhere else to receive the blessing of peaceful sleep. The full moon is not the only opportunity to nurture your dreams; seeding positive change is not reserved for the new moon. Every single night offers the hope of renewal. Rest assured that there is a ritual for every phase and season of your life.

Rituals are best learned one at a time to ensure your complete immersion and enjoyment. As you become more familiar with how certain rituals influence your being, you can experiment with pairing rituals to create a sequence that suits the season you're in. This is a creative act of self-advocacy (declaring what you need in order to feel whole and well) and deepens not only your ritual practice but also your understanding of yourself.

Performing the same set of rituals each night makes it physically easier to fall asleep, yet there will likely be times when you need more support in one area of your life than in others. Sometimes, all areas will seem to be in upheaval. Some nights you can go with the bare essentials; other nights will call for something magical. Sleep rituals are what *you* need them to be. Whether you have 3 minutes or 3 hours, establishing a solid evening practice gives you something to lean on in hard times.

Crafting a custom nighttime ritual sequence—that meets you where you are and leaves you feeling better than it found you—is an intuitive and kind endeavor. How you choose to design your night is entirely up to you and it is entirely okay to alter that design when you need to. Through your conscious, compassionate exploration, you will become more acquainted with your specific needs and more able to discern which rituals are ideal and will feel most supportive tonight.

To help you build a personalized ritual sequence that feels wholly of service tonight, spend a moment checking in with yourself:

1. With one hand on your forehead, ask: "How is my head?"
2. With hands on your heart, ask: "How is my heart?"
3. With one hand on your belly and the other on your low back, ask: "How is my vessel?"
4. With hands on each leg, ask: "How supported do I feel?"
5. With hands open to the sky, ask: "How open do I feel?"

Rather than seeking distinct or immediate answers to these questions, simply observe without judgment which area(s) attract your attention. Sensations that are noticeably more or less profound in any area could indicate an imbalance of some kind. Listen with your energy. Feel with your breath. Repeat as many times as you feel called to. Embrace your intuition, even if it's not as crystalline as you would like it to be: this is a stepping stone toward harmony. Your subtle inner inklings offer guidance like nothing else can and through these consultations you will grow a keen sensitivity to them.

Topics of interest that might come up include:

★ **MENTAL WELL-BEING**: Worry. Creativity. Yearning for change. Feeling stagnant. Boredom. Overwhelming responsibilities or possibilities. Setting goals. Loss of interest in work or career. Desire for knowledge.

★ **EMOTIONAL WELL-BEING**: Relationships with others and self. Loss. Sorrow. Shame. Attachments. Vulnerability (not necessarily a negative). Overwhelming social obligations and requests. Setting boundaries.

★ **PHYSICAL WELL-BEING**: Empowerment. Weakness. Loss of abilities or talent. Fatigue. Pain. Self-image. Sense of separateness.

★ **SPIRITUAL WELL-BEING**: Faith. Unconditional love. Forgiveness. Contentment. Connection to a greater power or plan. Intuition. Higher awareness. Reverence.

This moment of self-inquiry can help you select which rituals you feel a strong connection to tonight. While you may want to choose only one ritual from certain chapters (like Chapter 4), you can certainly choose more than one ritual from others. Consider how much time you can dedicate to tonight's practice and select anywhere from two to a "handful" of rituals that resonate with your innermost longings.

If you crave a touch more guidance as you're making your selections, you can pose a few questions to illuminate your most heartfelt "yeses":

1. Would this really feel nurturing to me?
2. Am I willing to be totally present for and in this practice?
3. Does this feel integral to my peace tonight (or can I save it for another night)?

Listen to the sensations that seem to be begging for a moment more of your time. Trust that whichever rituals you are positively drawn to are those that will best serve you tonight—mind, heart, body, and soul. Since each domain of life interacts with and affects the others, every ritual is capable of bestowing holistic support. Start with a simple pairing of two or three rituals and gradually grow from there. Move slowly and patiently as you craft a unique experience. Remember: this is not about filling your time; it is about filling your cup. It is about connection.

Below are two sample ritual sequences for those distressing seasons that call for a little extra support and an evening dedicated to solace.

WORRY NOT

A ritual sequence to soothe anxiety, fears, rumination, regretfulness, and intellectual exhaustion and open your mind to peaceful possibilities unfolding in your life:

1. Bee Breath (see Chapter 6)
2. Tapping for Peace (see Chapter 9)
3. Sage Smudging (see Chapter 2)
4. Magic Moon Dance (see Chapter 2)
5. Lavender Cherry Moon Milk (see Chapter 4)
6. Epsom Salt Foot Soak (see Chapter 3) while Pondering Inspirational Text (see Chapter 7)

7. Magnesium Oil Foot Massage (see Chapter 3)
8. Evening Pages (see Chapter 9)
9. Candle Gazing Meditation (see Chapter 7)
10. Sufi Grinding (see Chapter 5)
11. Reclining Abdominal Twist (see Chapter 5)
12. Legs Up the Wall (see Chapter 5) with a Botanical Dream Eye Pillow (see Chapter 3) and a selenite or celestite crystal
13. Optional, if you wake up: Shabad Kriya (see Chapter 6) or Choosing Your Dreams (see Chapter 8)

COMFORT AND CONSOLATION

A ritual sequence to soften depression, grief, loneliness, hopelessness, bitterness, and emotional exhaustion and open your heart to infinite healing guidance:

1. Diffusing Essential Oils (see Chapter 2): *Heart Constellations* or *Still Moments*
2. Luxurious Milk and Salt Bath (see Chapter 3) with rose petals and/or chamomile flowers
3. Self-Loving Oil Massage (see Chapter 3)
4. SerendipiTEA (see Chapter 4): *Comforts the heart* recipe; or add Rose Petal Infused Honey (see Chapter 4) to your tea
5. Healing Energy Blanket (see Chapter 8)
6. Letters from the Sky (see Chapter 9)
7. Child's Pose (see Chapter 5)
8. Bridge Pose (see Chapter 5)
9. Diaphragmatic Breathing (see Chapter 6) lying down with a rhodonite or rose quartz crystal

10. Yoga Nidra (see Chapter 7)

11. Lullaby Linen Mist (see Chapter 2): *Moon Moods* or *Peace Eternal*

12. Optional, right before bed or if you wake up: Left Nostril Breathing (see Chapter 6) or Visiting Your Happy Place (see Chapter 8)

As you navigate how you can best support yourself in this phase of life, you are not only learning to address imbalances and cope with stress more gracefully but you are learning to treat yourself differently.

Genuine care is closely related to compassion and is lovely when laced with patience and curiosity. Accessing these qualities through ritual is a balm for all kinds of suffering. Freed from the diversions of rejection—of yourself, others, life as it was and is—your evenings will begin to mirror the slow, successive rhythms of the seasons. In nature, everything happens in its own due time: dark and light, day and night. The slow and steady rhythms of your nightly rituals will naturally yield to the slow and steady rhythms of sleep. Enjoy the transition. Be in each season. You are honoring sleep and you are honoring yourself.

INDEX

Index

ABOUT THE AUTHOR

Jennifer Williamson is the creator of the online journal AimHappy.com, where she explores conscious living after loss through healing poetry, affirmation, and down-to-earth wisdom. Her first book, *Sleep Affirmations*, marked the beginning of a dream come true: making her work and love tangible in the world. Every composition is an offering of light and an invitation to shine. She lives in central Massachusetts.